LECTURE NOTES ON

Clinical
Anaesthesia

CARL L. GWINNUTT
MB, BS, MRCS, LRCP, FRCA
Consultant Anaesthetist
Hope Hospital, Salford

Honorary Clinical Lecturer in Anaesthesia
University of Manchester

FOREWORD BY
FRANK WALTERS

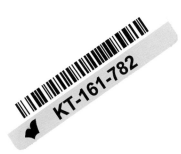

Blackwell
Science

© 1997 by Blackwell Science Ltd
a Blackwell Publishing Company

Editorial Offices:
Blackwell Science Ltd, 9600 Garsington Road, Oxford OX4 2DQ, UK
    Tel: +44 (0)1865 776868
Blackwell Publishing, Inc., 350 Main Street, Malden, MA 02148-5020, USA
    Tel: +1 781 388 8250
Blackwell Science Asia Pty, 550 Swanston Street, Carlton, Victoria 3053, Australia
    Tel: +61 (0)3 8359 1011

First published 1997
Reprinted 1998, 1999, 2000, 2001, 2002, 2003

Library of Congress Cataloging-in-Publication Data

Gwinnutt, Carl L.
    Lecture notes on clinical anaesthesia
  / Carl L. Gwinnutt.
        p.   cm.
    ISBN 0-86542-656-2
    1. Anesthesiology. I. Title.
  II. Title: Anaesthesia.
    [DNLM: 1. Anaesthesia.   2. Anesthetics
  –administration & dosage.
  WO 200 G9945L 1997]
  RD81.G843   1997
  617.9'6–DC21
  DNLM/DLC
  for Library of Congress   96-39563
                                                        CIP

ISBN 0-86542-656-2 (BSL)
ISBN 0-632-04157-9 (International edition)

A catalogue record for this title is available from the British Library

Set by Excel Typesetters, Hong Kong
Printed and bound in India using acid-free paper
by Replika Press Pvt. Ltd., Kundli 131 028

For further information on Blackwell Publishing, visit our website:
www.blackwellpublishing.com

Contents

Foreword

The knowledge and skills of anaesthetists extend beyond simply 'passing the gas'. Thus anaesthetists have much to teach medical students in the perioperative management of patients, intensive care management of chronic pain, and resuscitation. Dr Gwinnutt has significant experience in teaching and writing for those entering the specialty and is also an examiner at the Royal College of Anaesthetists. One of the benefits of anaesthetic teaching is that basic physiological and pharmacological facts can be underlined with a clinical demonstration. Dr Gwinnutt has used this teaching tool by introducing basic science and stressing its importance with clinical applications and examples.

Dr Gwinnutt has carefully considered the needs of medical students, which today are relatively limited and well established. He has resisted the temptation to cover every aspect of anaesthesia which may be considered important for those learning about the specialty. The reader is presented with a skilfully written text which is interesting and informative. The young medical student trying to assimilate large amounts of knowledge from many different areas will find this book full of useful information and easy to read.

Those whose appetites are successfully whetted by Dr Gwinnutt's writing and who wish to pursue a career in anaesthesia or need to have anaesthetic skills should read *Clinical Anaesthesia*, a text for beginners by the same author with more depth and breadth.

F.J.M. Walters
Frenchay Hospital, Bristol

Preface

Should medical students be taught anaesthesia?

I firmly believe that they should. Upon qualifying as doctors, they will face a variety of anaesthetic-related problems while caring for patients both pre- and postoperatively. Where better to learn the answers to these problems than from an anaesthetist. They will also be expected to participate as a member of the resuscitation team, for which skills learnt during an anaesthetic attachment are vital. In addition to these areas, medical students should be made aware that anaesthetists do more than provide the conditions under which surgery can be performed safely. We have been at the forefront of the development and running of intensive care units and more recently, the evolution of the Chronic Pain Relief Team and the establishment of acute pain relief services.

With this book I have tried to provide an introduction for medical students to the areas of anaesthesia they will encounter, and provide answers to the questions so often asked. At the same time I have endeavoured to provide some understanding of the range of current anaesthetic practice. I have not presumed to include all the knowledge that some students may require. As the title states, the contents of this book are intended as a skeleton on which I hope they will build, using the many excellent texts that are available. If, after reading this book, students feel motivated to learn by desire rather than need, I will have achieved my aim.

C.L.G.

Acknowledgements

I would like to express my sincere thanks to the following who have given freely of their time and expertise to help create this book:

Dr Richard Morgan, Dr Tony McCluskey and Dr Tim Johnson for the chapters on Postanaesthesia Care, An Introduction to Intensive Care, and Anaesthetists and Chronic Pain Relief, respectively.

The Department of Medical Illustration, Salford Royal Hospitals NHS Trust and Gillian Lee Illustrations for the photographs and illustrations.

Dr Frank Walters for his unending advice and patience with the manuscript.

Last but not least, Cath Jones at Blackwell Science for making such a good job of putting it all together.

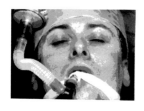

Anaesthetic Assessment and Premedication

The preoperative visit

> The preoperative visit of all patients by an anaesthetist is an essential requirement for the safe and successful conduct of anaesthesia

The main aim is to assess the patient's fitness for anaesthesia and there is no doubt that this is best performed by an anaesthetist, preferably the one who is going to administer the anaesthetic. The visit allows the most suitable anaesthetic technique to be determined, any potential interactions between concurrent diseases and anaesthesia anticipated, and finally provides an explanation and reassurance for the patient. Where there is coexisting illness, every opportunity must be taken to improve the patient's condition prior to surgery. This may mean seeking advice from other specialists to optimize treatment, although the final decision will rest with the anaesthetist. In an ideal world, all patients would be seen by their anaesthetist sufficiently ahead of the planned surgery to allow any problems identified to be treated without interfering with the smooth running of the operating list. For elective surgery, patients are rarely admitted more than 24 hours in advance and may not be seen by the anaesthetist until the evening prior to surgery. The anaesthetist frequently relies upon the junior surgical staff to ensure that all patients have a full history and examination so that during their visit they can concentrate on the areas of relevance to anaesthesia as detailed below.

There are three situations where special arrangements are usually made.

I *Patients with complex medical or surgical problems*. The patient is often admitted several days before surgery and the anaesthetist is actively involved in optimizing their condition prior to anaesthesia and surgery.

1

2 *Surgical emergencies.* Often only a few hours separates admission and operation in these patients. The anaesthetist must be informed as soon as the decision to operate has been made and their advice sought about the need for urgent investigations or treatment. This may occasionally mean delays in surgery, particularly if resuscitation is required.

3 *Day-case patients.* These are patients who are planned, non-resident admissions. They are generally 'fitter', having been selected specifically for this type of admission. Anaesthetic assessment is often carried out by the surgeon or a designated clinic nurse according to a protocol, and the patient's first contact with the anaesthetist is on arrival in the day-case unit. Some units run a preanaesthetic assessment clinic.

Anaesthetic history and examination

Ideally, the anaesthetist should take a full history and examine each patient, but for the reasons already identified this is seldom possible. This section concentrates on features of particular relevance to the anaesthetist.

PREVIOUS ANAESTHETICS AND OPERATIONS

These may have occurred in hospitals or dental surgeries. Enquire about inherited or 'family' diseases (e.g. sickle-cell disease, porphyria) and difficulties with previous anaesthetics (e.g. nausea, vomiting, dreams, awareness, postoperative jaundice). Check the records of previous anaesthetics to rule out or clarify problems such as difficulties with intubation, allergy to drugs administered, or adverse reactions (e.g. malignant hyperpyrexia, see below). The approximate date of previous anaesthetics, particularly if recent, should be identified to avoid the risk of repeat exposure to halothane (see page 59). Details of previous surgery may reveal potential anaesthetic problems, for example cardiac or pulmonary surgery.

PRESENT AND PAST MEDICAL HISTORY

Of all the aspects of the patient's medical history, those relating to the cardiovascular and respiratory systems are the most important. The questions and detail required will vary depending upon the disease present, its severity, anticipated anaesthesia and the planned operation.

Cardiovascular system

Specific enquiries must be made about:
- angina (its incidence, precipitating factors, duration, use of anti-anginal medications, e.g. glyceryl trinitrate (GTN) tablets or spray);
- previous myocardial infarction and subsequent symptoms;

- symptoms indicative of heart failure.

Patients with a proven history of myocardial infarction are at a greater risk of perioperative reinfarction, the incidence of which is related to the time interval between infarct and surgery. Elective surgery should be postponed until *at least* 6 months after the event. Untreated or poorly controlled hypertension (diastolic consistently >110 mmHg) may lead to exaggerated cardiovascular responses during anaesthesia. Both hypertension and hypotension can be precipitated which increase the risk of myocardial ischaemia. Heart failure will be worsened by the depressant effects of anaesthetic drugs on the heart, thereby impairing the perfusion of vital organs. Patients with valvular heart disease or who have prosthetic valves may be on anticoagulants. These may need to be stopped or changed prior to surgery. Antibiotic prophylaxis will be required during certain types of surgery.

Respiratory system

Enquire about symptoms related to:
- chronic obstructive lung disease, for example production of sputum (volume and colour);
- dyspnoea;
- asthma, including precipitating factors.

Patients with pre-existing lung disease are more prone to postoperative chest infections, particularly if they are also obese, or undergoing upper abdominal or thoracic surgery. If an acute upper respiratory tract infection (URTI) is present, anaesthesia and surgery should be postponed unless it is for a life-threatening condition. A patient's ability to perform everyday physical activities before having to stop because of symptoms (e.g. chest pain, shortness of breath) gives a very useful indication of both cardiac and respiratory reserve and can be assessed by asking questions such as:
- How far can you walk along the flat and uphill?
- Are you able to do housework or go shopping?
- How many stairs can you climb before stopping?
- Could you run for a bus?

Patients with severe musculoskeletal dysfunction (e.g. osteo- or rheumatoid arthritis) may not be able to exercise to the limit of their cardiorespiratory reserve.

Other conditions which are important if identified in the medical history

- *Indigestion, heartburn and reflux.* These may indicate the possibility of a hiatus hernia, which increases the risk of regurgitation and aspiration.

- *Rheumatoid disease.* Patients are often chronically anaemic and have severely limited movement of their joints which makes positioning for surgery and airway maintenance difficult.
- *Diabetes.* Patients have an increased incidence of ischaemic heart disease, renal dysfunction, and autonomic and peripheral neuropathy. These increase the incidence of intra- and postoperative complications, particularly infections.
- *Neuromuscular disorders.* Care must be taken when using muscle relaxants in these patients. Coexisting heart disease may be worsened by anaesthesia and restrictive pulmonary disease predisposes patients to postoperative chest infection.
- *Chronic renal failure.* Patients are usually anaemic, have electrolyte abnormalities and altered drug excretion, which restricts the choice of anaesthetic agents.
- *Jaundice.* This usually indicates infective or obstructive liver disease. Drug metabolism may be altered. The patient's coagulation must be checked preoperatively.
- *Epilepsy.* If well controlled, epilepsy is not a major problem but it is advisable to avoid anaesthetic agents which are potentially epileptogenic (e.g. enflurane, see page 60).

FAMILY HISTORY

All patients should be asked whether there are any known inherited conditions in the family or if any family members have ever experienced problems with anaesthesia. A history of prolonged apnoea after anaesthesia suggests pseudocholinesterase deficiency (see page 65) and an unexplained death suggests malignant hyperpyrexia (see below). Surgery should be postponed if any conditions are identified and the patient investigated appropriately. In the emergency situation, anaesthesia must be adjusted accordingly, for example avoidance of triggering agents in a patient with a family history of malignant hyperpyrexia.

DRUG HISTORY AND ALLERGIES

Identify all medications, both prescribed and self-administered. Patients will often forget about the oral contraceptive pill (OCP) and hormone replacement therapy (HRT), unless specifically asked. The incidence of use of medications rises with age and many of these drugs have important interactions with anaesthetics. The more common and important ones are listed at the end of this chapter (see Table 1.6). Allergies to drugs, topical preparations (e.g. iodine), adhesive dressings and foodstuffs should be noted.

SOCIAL HISTORY

- *Smoking.* Ascertain the number of cigarettes or the amount of tobacco smoked per day. Oxygen carriage is reduced by carboxyhaemoglobin and nicotine stimulates the sympathetic nervous system causing tachycardia, hypertension and coronary artery narrowing. Smokers have a significant increase in postoperative chest infections, chronic lung disease and carcinoma. Stopping smoking for 8 weeks improves the airways; for 2 weeks reduces their irritability; and for as little as 24 hours prior to anaesthesia decreases carboxyhaemoglobin levels.
- *Alcohol.* This is measured as units consumed per week, > 50 units/week causes induction of liver enzymes and tolerance to anaesthetic drugs. The risk of alcohol withdrawal syndrome postoperatively must be considered.
- *Drugs.* Ask specifically about the use of drugs for recreational purposes; including type, frequency and route of administration. This group of patients are at risk of infection with hepatitis B and human immunodeficiency virus (HIV). There can be difficulty with venous access in those using the intravenous (i.v.) route, due to widespread thrombosis of veins. Withdrawal syndromes can occur postoperatively.
- *Pregnancy.* The date of the last menstrual period should be noted in all women of childbearing age. Anaesthesia increases the risk of inducing a spontaneous abortion in early pregnancy. There is an increased risk of regurgitation and aspiration in late pregnancy. Elective surgery is best postponed until after delivery.

MALIGNANT HYPERPYREXIA

This is a rare inherited disorder of skeletal muscle metabolism, precipitated by exposure to certain anaesthetic drugs. The incidence varies, but may be between 1 : 10 000 and 1 : 40 000 anaesthetized patients. As the name suggests, the key feature is excess heat production causing a rise in core temperature of at least 2°C per hour. It occurs more commonly in patients undergoing certain operations, for example squint surgery, hernia repair, corrective orthopaedic surgery or cleft palate repair (see page 69).

THE EXAMINATION

As with the history that is taken, this concentrates on the cardiovascular and respiratory systems. Attention must also be paid to the airway, in order to try and identify those patients in whom there may be potential problems. The remaining systems are examined if problems relevant to anaesthesia are identified.

Cardiovascular system

Determine if there are any dysrhythmias, for example atrial fibrillation, and look for signs of heart failure. The presence of a heart murmur suggests valvular heart disease which may require further investigation. The patient's blood pressure is best measured at the end of the examination to try and eliminate the effect of anxiety. The peripheral veins should be inspected to identify any potential problems with i.v. access.

Respiratory system

Look for cyanosis, at the pattern of ventilation and count the respiratory rate. Dyspnoea may be present at rest. Wheeziness, signs of collapse, consolidation and effusion should be identified. The presence and degree of pulsus paradoxus is a useful indication of the severity of airway obstruction.

Nervous system

Chronic disease of the peripheral and central nervous systems should be identified and any evidence of motor or sensory impairment recorded. It must be remembered that some disorders will affect the cardiovascular and respiratory systems, for example dystrophia myotonica and multiple sclerosis.

Musculoskeletal

Patients with connective tissue disorders should have any restriction of movement and deformities noted. Patients suffering from chronic rheumatoid disease frequently have a reduced muscle mass, peripheral neuropathies and pulmonary involvement. Particular attention should be paid to the patient's cervical spine and temporomandibular joints (see below).

The airway

All patients must have an assessment made of their airway, the aim being to try and predict those patients who may be difficult to intubate. Assessment is often made in three stages.

I   *Observation of the patient's anatomy.*
  • Look for limitation of mouth opening, a receding mandible, position, number and health of teeth, size of tongue.
  • Examine the front of the neck for soft tissue swellings, deviated larynx or trachea.
  • Check the mobility of the cervical spine in both flexion and extension.

If any of these are abnormal, it suggests that intubation may be more difficult. However, it must be remembered that all of these are subjective.

2   *Simple bedside tests.*

• *Wilson score.* Increasing weight, a reduction in head and neck movement, mouth opening, and the presence of a receding mandible or buck teeth all predispose to increased difficulty with intubation.

• *Mallampati criteria.* The patient sitting upright is asked to open their mouth and maximally protrude their tongue. The view of the pharyngeal structures is noted and graded I–IV (Fig. 1.1). Grades III and IV suggest difficult intubation.

• *Thyromental distance.* With the head fully extended on the neck, the distance between the bony point of the chin and the prominence of the thyroid cartilage is measured (Fig. 1.2). A distance of less than 7 cm suggests difficult intubation.

3   *X-rays.* On a lateral X-ray of the head and neck, a reduced distance between the occiput and the spinous process of C1 (<5 mm) and an increase in the posterior depth of the mandible (>2.5 cm) suggest an impaired view at laryngoscopy. Allowance must be made for any magnification by the X-ray.

None of these tests, alone or in combination, predict all difficult intubations, but if problems are anticipated, anaesthesia should be planned accordingly. If intubation proves to be difficult, it must be recorded in a prominent place in the patient's notes and the patient informed.

Special investigations

There is little evidence to support the performance of 'routine' investigations. An investigation should only be ordered if the result of it will affect the way in which the patient will be managed. *In patients with no evidence of concurrent disease*, investigations can be limited as in Table 1.1.

ADDITIONAL INVESTIGATIONS

The following is a guide to those commonly requested.

• *Urea and electrolytes* — patients taking digoxin, diuretics, steroids and those with diabetes, renal disease, vomiting, diarrhoea.

• *Liver function tests* — patients with known hepatic disease, a history of a high alcohol intake (>50 units/week), with metastatic disease or evidence of malnutrition.

• *Blood sugar* — patients with diabetes, severe peripheral arterial disease or taking long-term steroids.

• *Electrocardiogram (ECG)* — patients known to be, or found to be, hypertensive or with symptoms or signs of heart disease.

MALLAMPATI ASSESSMENT

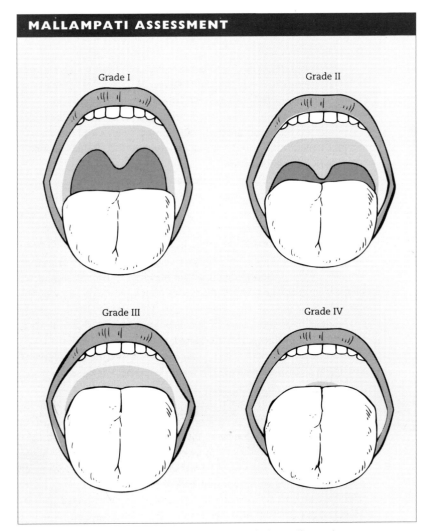

Fig. 1.1 The pharyngeal structures seen during Mallampati assessment.

- *Chest X-ray*—patients with a history or signs of cardiac or respiratory disease, suspected or known malignancy, where thoracic surgery is planned and in those patients from areas of endemic tuberculosis who have not had a chest X-ray in the last year.
- *Pulmonary function tests* — patients with dyspnoea on mild exertion, or who are asthmatic, require measurement of peak expiratory flow rate (PEFR), forced expiratory volume in 1 second (FEV_1) and forced

THYROMENTAL DISTANCE

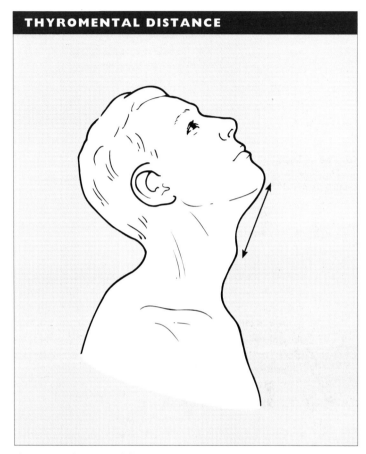

Fig. 1.2 The thyromental distance.

vital capacity (FVC). Patients who are dyspnoeic or cyanosed at rest, found to have an $FEV_1 < 60\%$ predicted, or are to have thoracic surgery, in addition to the above should have arterial blood gas analysed while breathing air.

• *Coagulation screen* — patients on anticoagulants, a history of a bleeding diatheses or a history of liver disease or jaundice.

• *Sickle-cell screen (Sickledex)* — patients with a family history of sickle-cell disease or where their ethnic origin puts them at risk of having sickle-cell disease. If positive, they may need electrophoresis for definitive diagnosis.

• *Cervical spine X-ray* — patients with rheumatoid arthritis, a history of major trauma or surgery to the neck, and those in whom difficult intubation is predicted.

BASELINE INVESTIGATIONS		
Age	Sex	Investigations
<40	Male	Nil
<40	Female	Hb
41–60	Male	ECG, blood sugar, serum creatinine
41–60	Female	Hb, ECG, blood sugar, creatinine
>61	All	Hb, ECG, blood sugar, creatinine
ECG, electrocardiogram; Hb, haemoglobin.		

Table 1.1 Baseline investigations for otherwise healthy patients.

Medical referral

Optimization of coexisting medical (or surgical) problems may mean postponing surgery and requesting the involvement of other specialists for advice about treatment. Physiotherapists as well as physicians play an important role in improving patients with respiratory problems, either as a result of pulmonary pathology (e.g. chronic obstructive lung disease) or secondary to neuromuscular or musculoskeletal disorders. Clearly a wide spectrum of conditions exist, the following are examples of some of the conditions more commonly encountered.

CARDIOVASCULAR DISEASE

- Untreated or poorly controlled hypertension or heart failure.
- Symptomatic ischaemic heart disease, despite treatment (unstable angina).
- Dysrhythmias: uncontrolled atrial fibrillation, paroxysmal supraventricular tachycardia, second and third degree heart block.
- The presence of congenital heart disease or symptomatic valvular heart disease.

RESPIRATORY DISEASE

- Chronic obstructive airways disease, particularly if dyspnoeic at rest.
- Bronchiectasis.
- Asthmatics who are unstable, taking oral steroids or have a $FEV_1 < 60\%$ predicted.

ENDOCRINE DISORDERS

- Insulin and non-insulin dependent diabetics who have ketonuria, glycated Hb $>10\%$ or a random blood sugar >12 mmol/l. Local policy will dictate referral of stable diabetics prior to surgery.

- Hypo- or hyperthyroidism symptomatic on current treatment.
- Cushing's or Addison's disease.
- Hypopituitarism.

RENAL DISEASE
- Chronic renal failure.
- Patients undergoing chronic dialysis.

HAEMATOLOGICAL DISORDERS
- Bleeding diatheses, for example haemophilia, thrombocytopenia.
- Therapeutic anticoagulation (including aspirin therapy).
- Haemoglobinopathies.
- Polycythaemia.
- Haemolytic anaemias.
- Leukaemias.

Risk assessment

Having assessed the patient preoperatively, it is not surprising that anaesthetists try to assess the risks of anaesthesia (and surgery). In the United Kingdom, the Confidential Enquiry into Perioperative Deaths (CEPOD, 1987) revealed an *overall* perioperative mortality of 0.7% in approximately 500 000 operations. Anaesthesia was considered to have been a contributing factor in 410 deaths, but judged *completely* responsible in only 3 cases — a primary mortality rate of 1:185 000 operations. When the deaths where anaesthesia contributed were analysed, the predominant factor was human error (Table 1.2). Although problems with equipment are often described, these were shown to be minimal.

SPECIAL INDICATORS
The leading cause of death after surgery is myocardial infarction and in addition there is significant morbidity from non-fatal infarction. Attempts

ANAESTHETIC ASSOCIATED DEATHS

Inadequate preoperative preparation including resuscitation
Lack of and inappropriate monitoring during surgery
Poor postoperative care, including lack of intensive care beds
Inadequate supervision of trainees
Out-of-hours operating

Table 1.2 Major factors identified as contributing to anaesthetic associated deaths.

INCREASED RISK OF MORTALITY

Increasing age: > 60 years
Sex: male > female
Worsening physical status
Increasing number of concurrent medical conditions, in particular:
   myocardial infarction
   diabetes mellitus
   renal disease
Increasing complexity of surgery:
   intracranial
   major vascular
   intrathoracic
Increasing length of surgery (> 2 hours)
Emergency operations

Table 1.3 Factors associated with increased risk of mortality.

ASA PHYSICAL STATUS SCALE

Class	Physical status
I	A healthy patient with no organic or psychological disease process. The pathological process for which operation is performed is localized and causes no systemic upset
II	A patient with a mild to moderate systemic disease process caused by the condition to be treated surgically or other pathological process which does not limit the patient's activities in any way, e.g. treated hypertensive, stable diabetic. Patients aged ≥ 80 years are automatically placed in class II
III	A patient with severe systemic disease from any cause which imposes a definite functional limitation on activity, e.g. ischaemic heart disease, chronic obstructive lung disease
IV	A patient with a severe systemic disease which is a constant threat to life, e.g. unstable angina
V	A moribund patient, unlikely to survive 24 hours with or without surgery

Note: 'E' may be added to signify an emergency operation.

Table 1.4 American Society of Anesthesiologists (ASA) physical status scale.

ASA STATUS AND POSTOPERATIVE MORTALITY		
ASA class	Absolute mortality (%)	Crude mortality per 10 000 anaesthetics
I	0.1	7.2
II	0.2	19.7
III	1.8	115.1
IV	7.8	766.2
V	9.4	3358.0

Table 1.5 Relationship between American Society of Anesthesiologists (ASA) status and postoperative mortality.

have been made to identify factors which will predict those patients at risk. One system used to predict the risk of a cardiac event is the Goldman index (see Further reading).

GENERAL INDICATORS

A wide variety of other factors have been identified as contributing to the risk of mortality in the operative and postoperative period (Table 1.3).

Of the factors listed in Table 1.3, physical status has proved to be a powerful predictor of postoperative mortality. The commonest method of categorizing patients is by using the American Society of Anesthesiologists (ASA) physical status scale (Table 1.4). The patient's ASA physical status has been shown to be related to both absolute and crude postoperative mortality (Table 1.5).

Further reductions in the perioperative mortality of patients have been shown to result from improving preoperative preparation by optimizing patient's physical status, adequately resuscitating those who require emergency surgery, appropriate monitoring intraoperatively and the provision of postoperative care, in a high dependency or intensive care unit if indicated.

Informing the patient

Often, the anaesthetist has only a brief time in which to develop a relationship with the patient and one of the most important things is to explain the events the patient will experience in the perioperative period, avoiding technical jargon, followed by an opportunity to ask questions.

Most patients will want to know how long they are to be starved prior to surgery, both in terms of eating and drinking. It is important that they are given clear instructions regarding the arrangements for taking their normal medications and whether they can have a small amount of water to take tablets. If a premedication is prescribed, the approximate timing, route of administration and likely effects should be discussed.

The choice of anaesthetic technique rests with the anaesthetist, but most patients appreciate some details of what to expect. The induction of general anaesthesia is most commonly achieved by an i.v. injection through an indwelling cannula, producing rapid loss of consciousness. If regional anaesthesia is used, it should be pointed out that remaining conscious throughout is to be expected unless some form of sedation is to be used. If large numbers of invasive monitoring devices are to be used prior to anaesthesia, the procedures should be described in such a way as to not alarm or frighten the patient.

Most patients will ask about their immediate recovery. For most, this will be in a recovery ward or a similar unit. It is advisable to warn about the possibility of drains, catheters and drips as their presence may be misinterpreted by the patient as indicating unexpected problems. Where postoperative care is planned to take place in the intensive care unit, the patient should be told what to expect and, if at all possible, be given the opportunity to visit the unit a few days before and meet some of the staff.

Finally, it is important to reassure patients about postoperative pain control. They will need to be informed of the technique to be used, particularly if it requires their co-operation, for example a patient-controlled analgesia device (see page 122).

As consent for anaesthesia becomes a separate entity (currently it is included in the consent for surgery), the information given to the patient and the time this takes is likely to increase in order that consent is truly informed.

Premedication

Premedication originally referred to drugs administered to facilitate the induction and maintenance of anaesthesia (literally, preliminary medication). Nowadays, premedication refers to the administration of any drugs in the period prior to induction of anaesthesia. Consequently, a wide variety of drugs are used with a variety of aims.

> **The 6 As of premedication**
> Anxiolysis
> Amnesia
> Anti-emetic
> Antacid
> Anti-autonomic
> Analgesic

ANXIOLYSIS

The most commonly prescribed drugs are the benzodiazepines. They produce a degree of sedation and amnesia, are well absorbed from the gastrointestinal tract and are usually given orally, 45–90 minutes preoperatively. Those most commonly used include temazepam 20–30 mg, diazepam 10–20 mg and lorazepam 2–4 mg.

Other agents include phenothiazines (promazine), antihistamines (promethazine, trimeprazine) and β-blockers in patients who suffer from excessive somatic manifestations of anxiety, for example tachycardia. A preoperative visit and explanation is often as effective as drugs at alleviating anxiety and sedation does not always mean lack of anxiety.

AMNESIA

Some patients specifically request that they do not wish to have any recall of the events leading up to anaesthesia and surgery. This is usually accomplished by the administration of lorazepam which will provide anterograde amnesia.

ANTI-EMETIC (REDUCTION OF NAUSEA AND VOMITING)

Nausea and vomiting may follow the administration of opioids either pre- or intraoperatively. Certain types of surgery are associated with a higher incidence of postoperative nausea and vomiting, for example gynaecology. Drugs with useful anti-emetic properties include:

* dopamine antagonists, for example metoclopramide, domperidone, droperidol;
* antihistamines, for example cyclizine, promethazine;
* anticholinergics, for example atropine, hyoscine;
* phenothiazines, for example promazine;
* 5-hydroxytryptamine antagonists, for example ondansetron.

ANTACID (MODIFY pH AND VOLUME OF GASTRIC CONTENTS)

Patients are starved preoperatively to reduce the risk of regurgitation and aspiration of gastric acid. Patients who have received opiates preoperatively or present as emergencies, particularly if in pain, will have delayed gastric emptying and those with a hiatus hernia are at an increased risk of regurgitation. A variety of drug combinations are used to try and increase the pH and reduce the volume.

• Oral sodium citrate: chemically neutralizes residual acid.
• Cimetidine, ranitidine (H_2 antagonists): reduce acid secretion.
• Metoclopramide: increases gastric emptying and lowers oesophageal sphincter tone. This reduces the potential for regurgitation.

An alternative is aspiration of gastric contents via a naso- or orogastric tube.

ANTI-AUTONOMIC (BLOCK AUTONOMIC REFLEXES)

Parasympathetic reflexes

Excessive vagal activity, causing profound bradycardias, may be seen following:

• halothane, particularly when used for induction;
• repeated doses of suxamethonium;
• surgery, during traction on the extraocular muscles (squint correction), handling of the viscera or during elevation of a fractured zygoma.

The anticholinergic agents atropine and glycopyrrolate are used to protect against the occurrence of bradycardias and although used preoperatively they are most effective when administered intravenously at induction. They are also used to prevent excessive secretion of saliva associated with the presence of objects in the mouth, for example an oropharyngeal airway.

Sympathetic reflexes

Increased sympathetic activity can be seen at intubation causing tachycardia and hypertension. This is undesirable in certain patients, for example those with ischaemic heart disease or raised intracranial pressure. These responses can be attenuated by the use of β-blockers administered orally preoperatively (e.g. atenolol) or intravenously at induction (e.g. esmolol). An alternative is to administer potent analgesics at induction of anaesthesia, for example fentanyl or alfentanil.

ANALGESIA

Although the oldest form of premedication, analgesic drugs are now

MEDICATIONS AND ANAESTHETIC AGENTS

Drug group	Comments
1 Angiotensin-converting enzyme (ACE) inhibitors: Captopril Enalapril	Potent vasodilators. Synergistic with the effects of anaesthetics causing hypotension
2 Antibiotics: Aminoglycosides Polymixins	Synergistic with neuromuscular blocking drugs prolonging length of block. Renal toxicity with long-term therapy or combination with some diuretics
3 Anticoagulants: (a) Oral: warfarin, nicoumalone (b) IV: heparin	Increased risk of haemorrhage during intubation, insertion of central lines, local/regional anaesthesia, *surgery*, insertion of a nasogastric tube
4 Anticonvulsants: Barbiturates Phenytoin Carbamazepine	Potent inducers of hepatic enzymes, may need increased doses of induction agents and opioids
5 Benzodiazepines	Wide variety of drugs with varying half-lives. Tolerance common. Additive effect with other CNS depressants. A withdrawal syndrome may be precipitated if flumazenil, a specific benzodiazepine antagonist, is administered
6 β-blockers: Atenolol Metoprolol Oxprenolol Propranolol Sotalol and others	Negative inotropic effects may combine with vasodilatation caused by anaesthetic agents to produce hypotension. The pulse rate is a poor guide to blood loss intraoperatively
7 Calcium antagonists: Diltiazem Nifedipine Verapamil	Isoflurane, enflurane and halothane are non-specific calcium antagonists. Effects additive, producing hypotension. Verapamil may cause bradycardias secondary to decreased atrioventricular conduction
8 Digoxin	Toxicity common, predisposing to arrhythmias, potentiated by suxamethonium
9 Diuretics: Thiazides Loop diuretics	Hypokalaemia causing dysrhythmias and prolonging neuromuscular blockade. Hyponatraemia

Table 1.6 (*Above and page 18*) Medications which may have an interaction with anaesthetic agents.

MEDICATIONS AND ANAESTHETIC AGENTS

Drug group	Comments
10 Lithium	Prolongs the effects of non-depolarizing neuromuscular blocking drugs
11 Monoamine oxidase inhibitors (MAOIs): Isocarboxazid Phenelzine Tranylcypromine	Uncommon but potentially fatal interactions with opioids, particularly pethidine, and all sympathomimetics. Must be stopped at least 2 weeks before surgery
12 Steroids	Hypotension at induction of anaesthesia. Supplementary doses required for patients on long-term treatment or if taken in the past 3 months, due to adrenocortical suppression
13 Tricyclic antidepressants	Potentiate the effects of exogenous catecholamines causing arrhythmias, e.g. adrenaline, when it is used as a vasoconstrictor in local anaesthetics or to reduce bleeding

CNS, central nervous system.

Table 1.6 *Continued*

generally reserved for patients who are in pain preoperatively and they are usually administered intramuscularly. The most commonly used are morphine, pethidine and fentanyl. Morphine was widely used for its sedative effects but is relatively poor as an anxiolytic and has largely been replaced by the benzodiazepines. In addition, opiates have a range of unwanted side-effects including, nausea, vomiting, respiratory depression and delayed gastric emptying.

MISCELLANEOUS

A variety of other drugs are commonly administered prophylactically prior to anaesthesia and surgery, for example:
- steroids: to patients on long-term treatment or who have received them within the past 3 months;
- antibiotics: to patients with prosthetic or diseased heart valves, or undergoing joint replacement;
- anticoagulants: as prophylaxis against deep venous thrombosis;
- transdermal GTN: either as patches or a paste (Percutol) in patients with ischaemic heart disease to reduce the risk of coronary ischaemia;

- Eutectic mixture of local anaesthetics (EMLA): a topically applied local anaesthetic cream to reduce the pain of inserting an i.v. cannula.

In addition to these are the patient's own regular medications, which should be taken as instructed by the anaesthetist (Table 1.6).

Further reading

Buck N, Devlin HB, Lunn JN. *The Report of a Confidential Enquiry into Perioperative Deaths.* London: Nuffield Provincial Hospitals Trust, 1987.

Cobly M, Vaughan RS. Recognition and management of difficult airway problems. *British Journal of Anaesthesia* 1992; **68**: 90–7.

Cohen MM, Duncan PG, Tate RB. Does anesthesia contribute to operative mortality? *Journal of the American Medical Association* 1988; **260** (19): 2859–63.

Frerk CM. Predicting difficult intubation. *Anaesthesia* 1991; **46**: 1005–8.

Goldman L, Calder DL, Nussbaum SR *et al.* Multifactorial index of cardiac risk in noncardiac surgical procedures. *New England Journal of Medicine* 1977; **297**: 845–9.

Mamode N, Cobbe S, Pollock JG. Infarcts after surgery. *British Medical Journal* 1995; **310**: 1215–16.

Vacanti CJ, VanHouten RJ, Hill RC. A statistical analysis of the relationship of physical status to postoperative mortality in 68 388 cases. *Anesthesia and Analgesia* 1970; **49** (4): 564–6.

Wilson ME, Speiglhalter D, Robertson, JA *et al.* Predicting difficult intubation. *British Journal of Anaesthesia* 1988; **61**: 211–16.

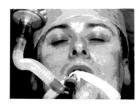

The Delivery of Anaesthetic Gases and Vapours

Anaesthesia is usually induced by an intravenous (i.v.) injection and then maintained by the administration of gases and vapours. Although the term 'anaesthetic gases' is widely used, strictly speaking nitrous oxide and carbon dioxide are vapours, as they are liquids at the temperature and pressure they are stored under. In order to avoid confusion, the term 'vapours' will only be used in reference to the volatile anaesthetic agents.

The delivery of gases to the operating theatre

Most hospitals now use a piped medical gas and vacuum system (PMGV) to distribute oxygen, nitrous oxide, medical air and vacuum. The distribution pipelines end in outlets which act as self-closing sockets, each specifically coloured and labelled for one gas. Onward delivery to the anaesthetic machine is via flexible reinforced hoses, colour coded throughout their length, which attach to the wall outlet by a removable gas-specific probe (Fig. 2.1) and to the anaesthetic machine via a gas-specific nut and union. Cylinders, which were the traditional method of supplying gases to the anaesthetic machine, are now mainly used as reserves in case of pipeline failure. Commonly used medical gases and cylinder sizes are shown in Table 2.1.

OXYGEN

Piped oxygen is supplied from a liquid oxygen reserve, where it is stored under pressure (10–12 bar, 1200 kPa) at approximately −180°C in a vacuum insulated evaporator (VIE), effectively a Thermos flask. Gaseous oxygen is removed from above the liquid, or by vaporizing liquid oxygen using heat from the environment. The gas is warmed to ambient air temperature en route from the VIE to the pipeline system. A reserve bank of

MEDICAL GAS CYLINDERS

	Size						Colour	
	C	D	E	F	G	J	Body	Shoulder
Oxygen	170	340	680	1360	3400	6800	Black	White
Nitrous oxide	450	900	1800	3600	9000	—	Blue	Blue
Entonox	—	500	—	2000	5000	—	Blue	Blue/white
Air	—	—	640	1280	3200	6400	Grey	White/black
Carbon dioxide	450	—	1800	3600	—	—	Grey	Grey

Table 2.1 Medical gas cylinder sizes, contents (l) and colours.

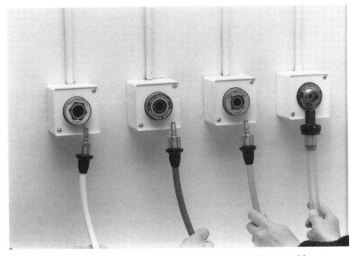

Fig. 2.1 Wall-mounted outlets for (left to right) oxygen, nitrous oxide, vacuum and scavenging, and gas-specific probes and hoses.

cylinders of compressed oxygen is kept adjacent in case of failure of the main system.

Oxygen in cylinders is stored at 12 000 kPa (120 bar, 1980 pounds per square inch (psi)) above its critical temperature (−118°C) and is therefore in the gaseous state. If the volume in a full cylinder is known, the contents at any time can be estimated from the cylinder pressure by using the ideal gas equation.

NITROUS OXIDE

Piped nitrous oxide is supplied from large (G size) cylinders, several of which are joined together to form a bank and attached to a common manifold. There are usually two banks, one which is running (duty bank) with all cylinders turned on, and a reserve bank. In addition, there is a small emergency supply. Smaller cylinders are attached directly to the anaesthetic machine (D and E sizes).

Nitrous oxide is stored at 440 kPa (640 psi) and at room temperature ($\approx 20°C$) is below its critical temperature (36.4°C) and is therefore liquid within the cylinder. If the weight of an empty cylinder is known, then an estimate of the contents can be made by weighing it. The pressure in the cylinder cannot be used as this stays constant while any liquid remains, providing that the temperature of the liquid remains constant. In reality, some drop in pressure does occur due to cooling of the liquid and gas as a result of providing the latent heat of vaporization. When all the liquid has evaporated, the cylinder contains only gas, and as it empties, the pressure falls rapidly to zero.

MEDICAL AIR

This is supplied either by the use of a compressor or in cylinders. A compressor delivers air to a central reservoir, where it is dried and filtered to achieve the desired quality before distribution. It is supplied in cylinders at 13 700 kPa (2000 psi), and via the pipeline system for anaesthetic use at 400 kPa (60 psi) and at 700 kPa (100 psi) to power medical tools.

VACUUM

The final part of the PMGV system is medical vacuum. Two pumps are connected to a system which must be capable of generating a vacuum of at least 400 mmHg below atmospheric pressure. This is delivered to the anaesthetic rooms, operating theatre and other appropriate sites. At several stages between the outlets and the pumps there are drains and bacterial filters to prevent contamination by aspirated fluids.

The anaesthetic machine

This is often referred to as the 'Boyle's machine', its main functions are:
• to reduce the pressure of the gases from the pipelines or cylinders to a level safe for use with patients;
• to allow the accurate delivery of varying flows of gases to a patient breathing system;
• to allow additional anaesthetic vapours to be added to the gas stream.

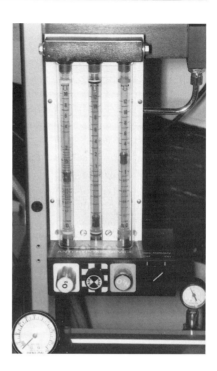

Fig. 2.2 Oxygen, air and nitrous oxide flowmeters. Note the presence of an antihypoxic device.

REDUCTION OF GAS PRESSURE

Cylinder gases must first pass through a regulating or reducing valve which reduces the pressure to 400 kPa (60 psi) before onward transmission to the flowmeters (see below). The piped gases are already at 400 kPa and therefore need no further reduction prior to reaching the flowmeters.

MEASUREMENT OF FLOW

This is achieved on most anaesthetic machines by the use of flowmeters ('rotameters'; Fig. 2.2) which have the following features:
- A specific calibrated flowmeter is required for each gas.
- A rotating bobbin floats in the gas stream, its upper edge indicating the rate of gas flow.
- Several flowmeters are mounted together on the left-hand side of the anaesthetic machine, oxygen being at the extreme left edge.
- The control for oxygen has a different knurled finish and is usually more prominent.
- Flowmeters do not regulate pressure.

Points to note

• Leakage from the oxygen flowmeter will result in a hypoxic mixture as it is the most upstream gas. On modern machines oxygen enters downstream to the other gases to prevent this.

• As all gases have independent flow controls, accidental delivery of a hypoxic mixture to the patient is possible. Newer anaesthetic machines have a system whereby the oxygen and nitrous oxide controls are linked such that <25% oxygen cannot be delivered (see Fig. 2.2). In addition, the flow of carbon dioxide may be limited to 500 ml/minute.

Safety features on anaesthetic machines

1 An emergency oxygen 'flush' device can be used to deliver pure oxygen at 35 l/minute minimum.

2 A non-return valve is used to minimize the effects of back pressure on the function of flowmeters and vaporizers.

3 An alarm to warn of oxygen failure, usually audible and driven either by the failing oxygen supply or the nitrous oxide. Some devices also discontinue the nitrous oxide supply and if the patient is breathing spontaneously, allow them to entrain air.

THE ADDITION OF ANAESTHETIC VAPOURS

Agent-specific vaporizers are used to produce an accurate concentration of each inhalational agent:

• modern vaporizers produce a saturated vapour from a reservoir of liquid anaesthetic;

• wicks increase the surface area from which vaporization can take place;

• the final concentration of anaesthetic agent is controlled by varying the proportion of gas passing into the vapour chamber;

• the vaporizers are **te**mperature **c**ompensated (hence -tec suffix, e.g. Fluotec) to account for the loss of latent heat which causes cooling and reduces vaporization of the anaesthetic.

The resultant mixture of gases and vapour is finally delivered to a common outlet on the anaesthetic machine. From this point, specialized breathing systems are used to transfer the gases and vapours to the patient.

CHECKING THE ANAESTHETIC MACHINE

In the anaesthetic room patients are rendered unconscious, deprived of their protective reflexes and they may be made apnoeic. It is essential that the anaesthetist is both confident and competent at using the equipment at their disposal, in particular the anaesthetic machine, to ensure that the patient suffers no harm. It is the responsibility of each anaesthetist to ensure that the apparatus used will function in the manner expected. The main danger is that the anaesthetic machine appears to perform normally, but in fact is delivering a hypoxic mixture to the patient. In order to minimize the risk of this, the Association of Anaesthetists of Great Britain and Ireland have published a *Checklist for Anaesthetic Machines*. Its main aims are to ensure that oxygen flows through the oxygen delivery system and is unaffected by the use of any additional gas or vapour. It is recommended that this check is performed at the beginning of each operating session and is the responsibility of the anaesthetist.

Anaesthetic breathing systems

In spontaneously breathing patients, gases travel from the anaesthetic machine via an 'anaesthetic circuit', or more correctly an anaesthetic breathing system. Contact with the patient is made via a facemask, laryngeal mask or tracheal tube (see Chapter 3). There are five basic systems, referred to as 'Mapleson A, B, C, D or E', after their classification by W.W. Mapleson, and some carry the names of their inventors. Because several patients in succession may breathe through the same system, it is becoming increasingly common to place a low-resistance, disposable, bacterial filter at the patient end of the system. This is changed between patients to reduce the risk of cross-infection.

COMPONENTS OF A BREATHING SYSTEM

All systems consist of the following:

• *A connection for fresh gas input:* usually the common gas outlet on the anaesthetic machine, or via small bore tubing close to the patient.

• *A reservoir bag:* usually of 2 l capacity to allow the patient's peak inspiratory demands (30–40 l/minute) to be met with a lower constant flow from the anaesthetic machine (6–8 l/minute). Its excursion gives an indication of ventilation, and allows manual ventilation of the patient. It also acts as a further safety device being easily distended at low pressure if obstruction occurs.

• *An adjustable expiratory valve:* to vent expired gas, eliminating carbon dioxide. During spontaneous ventilation, resistance to opening is minimal so as not to impede expiration. Closing the valve allows manual ventilation by squeezing the reservoir bag.

The following sections give a brief description of the systems used; those wishing further details should consult Further reading at the end of the chapter.

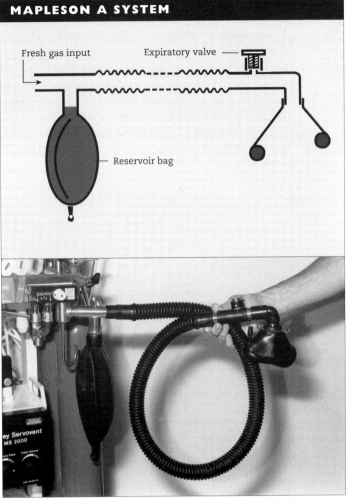

Fig. 2.3 Diagram of the Mapleson A system and photograph of the system connected to the common gas outlet on the anaesthetic machine.

Mapleson A or Magill (Fig. 2.3)

This is efficient for use with spontaneous ventilation, providing there are no leaks. A fresh gas flow of 5–6 l/minute in a 70 kg adult (equivalent to the patient's alveolar minute ventilation) will prevent rebreathing of carbon dioxide.

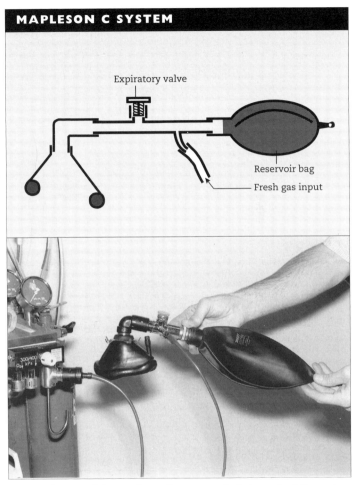

MAPLESON C SYSTEM

Expiratory valve

Reservoir bag

Fresh gas input

Fig. 2.4 Diagram of the Mapleson C system and photograph of the system connected to the gas outlet on the anaesthetic machine.

Mapleson C or Westminster facepiece (Fig. 2.4)

In this system, the gas inflow is via a small diameter side port, adjacent to the expiratory valve. Its compactness makes it useful during resuscitation or transportation. However, it is inefficient for use in both spontaneous and controlled ventilation as it requires a fresh gas flow of 12–14 l/minute to prevent rebreathing of carbon dioxide. In inexperienced

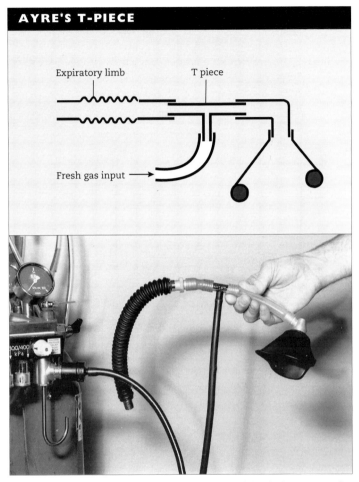

Fig. 2.5 Diagram of Ayre's T-piece and photograph of the device connected to an anaesthetic machine.

hands the use of a self-inflating bag with a non-rebreathing valve is preferable during resuscitation.

Mapleson E or Ayre's T-piece (Fig. 2.5)

This is a T-shaped device. The fresh gas inflow is via one limb, connection to a facemask or tracheal tube via the second and the third limb acts as a reservoir and allows venting of expired and excess gas. The lack of an expiratory valve helps to keep resistance to expiration minimal and this system has been widely used in paediatric anaesthesia.

The Bain system (modification of the Mapleson D system) (Fig. 2.6)

Fresh gas inflow is at the patient end of the system via the central small bore tube. This is a very efficient system during controlled ventilation, a fresh gas flow equal to the patient's minute volume (or 70 ml/kg) maintaining normocarbia.

NB. If the inner tube becomes disconnected the patient will simply rebreath expired gas and rapidly become hypoxic and hypercarbic.

THE CIRCLE SYSTEM

The anaesthetic breathing systems described so far have relied on a combination of the opening of an expiratory valve and the inflow of fresh anaesthetic gas to eliminate carbon dioxide. Even the most efficient system is still wasteful as the expired gas contains oxygen and anaesthetic agents as well as carbon dioxide. The circle system (Fig. 2.7) overcomes these inefficiencies as follows:

• The expired gases are passed through a container of soda lime (the absorber), which is a mixture of calcium, sodium and potassium hydroxide, to chemically remove carbon dioxide.

• Supplementary oxygen and anaesthetic agents are added to maintain the desired concentrations, and the gases are rebreathed by the patient. The circle system is therefore the only true 'anaesthetic circuit'.

• The gases are warmed and humidified as they pass through the absorber (by-products of the reaction removing carbon dioxide).

There are several points of note when using a circle system.

• The exact concentration of oxygen within the circle is not known and the inspired concentration must be monitored to ensure that the patient is not rendered hypoxic (see Chapter 5).

• The inspired anaesthetic concentration must be monitored, particularly when a patient is being ventilated through a circle, to prevent awareness.

• When unable to absorb any more carbon dioxide, a change in the colour of the granules occurs as a result of the incorporation of an indicator. One of the commonly used preparations changes from pink to white.

Mechanical ventilation

A wide variety of anaesthetic ventilators are available, each of which

BAIN SYSTEM

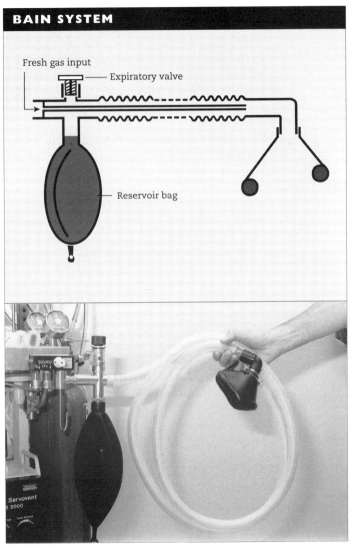

Fresh gas input

Expiratory valve

Reservoir bag

Fig. 2.6 Diagram and photograph of a Bain system connected to the gas outlet on the anaesthetic machine.

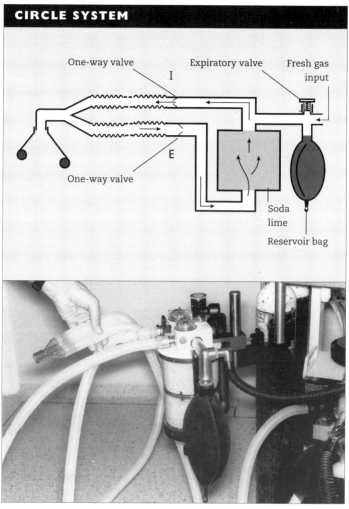

CIRCLE SYSTEM

One-way valve   Expiratory valve   Fresh gas input

I

One-way valve

E

Soda lime

Reservoir bag

Fig. 2.7 Diagram and photograph of the circle system. Note the unidirectional valves (I, inspiratory; E, expiratory) situated on the top of the absorber, and the fresh gas input via the small corrugated tubing adjacent to the reservoir bag.

functions in a slightly different way. It is beyond the remit of this book to describe each in detail and only an outline of the principles of mechanical ventilation are given. The interested reader should consult Further reading at the end of the chapter.

PRINCIPLES OF MECHANICAL VENTILATION

During mechanical ventilation, the ventilator applies a positive pressure to the anaesthetic gases to overcome airway resistance and elastic recoil of the chest, and flow occurs into the lungs (compare this to spontaneous ventilation where a negative intrathoracic pressure draws air in). This technique is usually referred to as *intermittent positive pressure ventilation* (IPPV). In both spontaneous and mechanical ventilation, expiration occurs by passive recoil of the lungs and chest wall. In order to generate a positive pressure, the ventilator requires a source of energy. This is usually either gravity or gas pressure.

Gravity

The Manley is a typical example of a ventilator using this operating principle. Gas from the anaesthetic machine collects within a bellows which is compressed by a weight and at a predetermined time a valve opens and the contents of the bellows are delivered to the patient (Fig. 2.8).

Gas pressure

There are many types of ventilator which utilize this principle. Gas from the anaesthetic machine collects in a bellows or bag situated in a rigid container (Fig. 2.9). The ventilator controls the delivery of a gas (usually oxygen) at high pressure into the container to compress the bellows or bag, delivering the contents to the patient. This system is often called a 'bag-in-bottle' ventilator.

THE EFFECTS OF POSITIVE PRESSURE VENTILATION

Respiratory system

- There is an increase in both the ratio of physiological dead space to tidal volume (V_D/V_T), and ventilation/perfusion (V/Q) mismatch, both of which impair oxygenation. An inspired oxygen concentration of around 30% is used to compensate for these effects and prevent hypoxaemia.
- The partial pressure of carbon dioxide (Pa_{CO_2}) is dependent on alveolar ventilation. There is a tendency to overventilate patients resulting in hypocarbia. This causes a respiratory alkalosis which 'shifts' the oxyhaemoglobin dissociation curve to the left, increasing the affinity of haemoglobin for oxygen, and thereby reducing offloading at the tissues. Severe hypocarbia will induce vasoconstriction in many organs including the brain and heart, thereby reducing blood flow, which may cause ischaemia and impaired function.

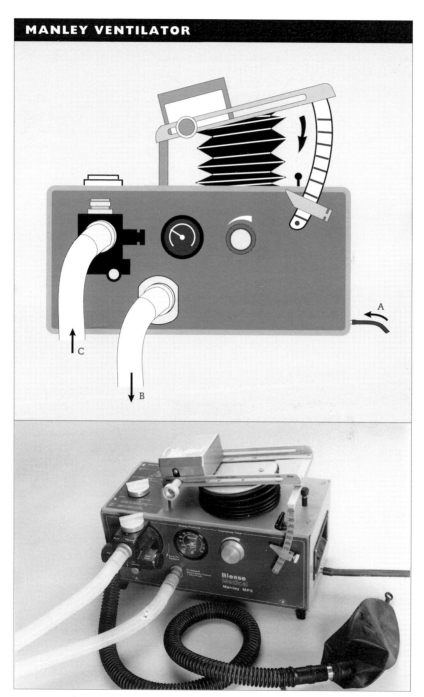

Fig. 2.8 Diagram and photograph of a gravity-powered ventilator. A, anaesthetic gas input; B, anaesthetic gas output to patient; C, expired gas from patient.

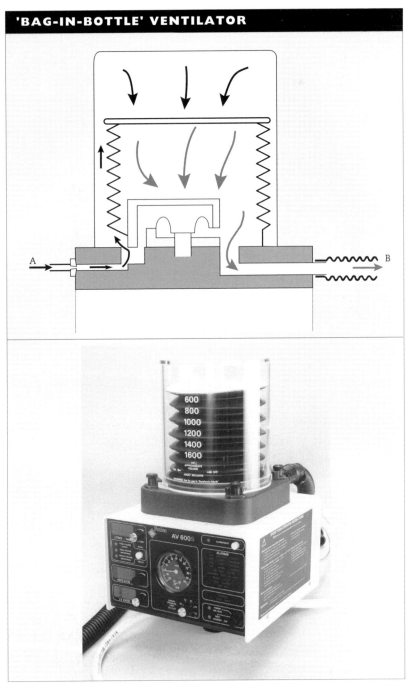

Fig. 2.9 Photograph and diagram of gas-powered ventilator ('bag-in-bottle'). A, high-pressure driving gas input; B, anaesthetic gas output to patient.

- Excessive positive pressure applied to the lungs may cause barotrauma, particularly in those patients with pre-existing lung disease.

Cardiovascular system

- The positive intrathoracic pressure reduces venous return to the heart and consequently cardiac output.
- Both systemic and pulmonary blood flow are reduced, the latter further increasing V/Q mismatch.
- The cardiac output is also reduced by hypocarbia causing vasoconstriction and increased peripheral vascular resistance.

SCAVENGING SYSTEMS

All the breathing systems described and mechanical ventilators, apart from the totally closed system, will vent varying volumes of excess and expired gas into the atmosphere immediately adjacent to the theatre staff. Although no conclusive evidence exists to link prolonged exposure to low concentrations of anaesthetic agents with any risks, it would seem sensible to minimize the degree of pollution within the operating theatre environment. Two types of scavenging systems are used as described below.

Passive systems

Gases from the expiratory valve are diverted to the outside atmosphere by the patient's expiratory effort. Consequently the resistance offered by the tubing used must be minimal, which limits its length. An alternative is to pass the gases through activated charcoal (The Cardiff Aldasorber). This removes volatile agents but not nitrous oxide.

Active systems

A low negative pressure is applied to the expiratory valve of the breathing system or ventilator to remove gases to the outside environment. A high flow is used and the patient protected against excessive negative pressure being applied to the lungs by valves with very low opening pressures.

The use of such systems does not eliminate the problem of pollution, it merely shifts it from one site to another. Anaesthetic agents, particularly nitrous oxide, are potent destroyers of ozone thereby adding to the 'greenhouse' effect. The use of circle systems, total i.v. and regional anaesthesia have a major role to play in the overall reduction of pollution by anaesthetic agents.

Further reading

Aitkenhead A, Smith G (eds). *Textbook of Anaesthesia,* 2nd edn. Edinburgh: Churchill Livingstone, 1990.

Daley A, Moyle JTB, Ward CS. *Ward's Anaesthetic Equipment,* 3rd edn. London: Saunders, 1992.

Mushin WW, Rendell-Baker L, Thompson PW, Mapleson WW. *Automatic Ventilation of the Lungs,* 3rd edn. Oxford: Blackwell Scientific Publications, 1980.

Scurr C, Feldman S, Soni N (eds). *Scientific Foundations of Anaesthesia,* 4th edn. Oxford: Heinemann Medical Books, 1990.

Wilkinson DJ. Evolution of the anaesthetic machine. *Current Anaesthesia and Critical Care* 1991; **2** (1): 51–6.

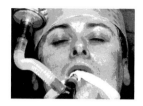

Managing the Airway

Maintenance of a patent airway is an essential prerequisite for the safe and successful conduct of anaesthesia. In addition, during resuscitation patients often have an obstructed airway either as the cause or result of their loss of consciousness. The skill of airway maintenance should be acquired by all doctors, and not simply regarded as the responsibility of the anaesthetist. The descriptions of airway management techniques which follow are intended to *supplement* practice either on a mannikin or preferably on an anaesthetized patient under the direction of a skilled anaesthetist.

Basic techniques

Anaesthesia frequently results in loss of the airway and it is most easily restored by a combination of the head tilt along with a jaw thrust (see Chapter 11). The latter is provided by the anaesthetist's fourth and fifth fingers (of one or both hands) lifting the angle of the mandible. The overall effect desired is that the patient's mandible is 'lifted' into the mask rather than the mask being pushed into the face (Fig. 3.1).

FACEMASKS

- The most commonly used type in adults is the BOC anatomical face-mask (Fig. 3.2) which is designed to fit the contours of the face with the minimum of pressure.
- Leakage of anaesthetic gases is minimized by an air-filled cuff around the edge.
- Masks are made in a variety of sizes and the smallest one which provides a good seal should be used (to minimize the increase in dead space which occurs).

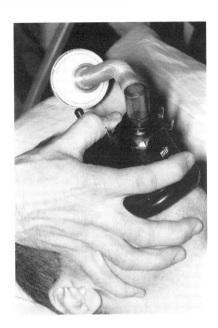

Fig. 3.1 Mask being held on patient's face.

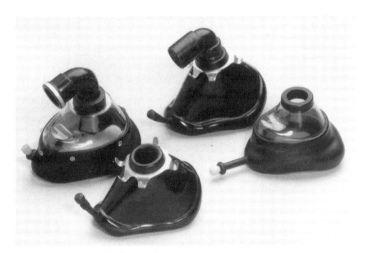

Fig. 3.2 BOC and Ambu facemasks.

- The Ambu mask (Fig. 3.2) has a transparent body—allowing identification of vomit—making it popular for resuscitation.
- All masks must be disinfected between each patient.

Simple adjuncts

The most commonly used are the oropharyngeal (Guedel) and nasopharyngeal airways, inserted after the induction of anaesthesia to help maintain the airway in conjunction with the techniques described above.

OROPHARYNGEAL AIRWAY

• These are curved plastic tubes, flattened in cross-section and flanged at the oral end, which lie over the tongue, preventing it from falling back into the pharynx.

• They are available in a variety of sizes from neonates to large adults. The commonest sizes are 2–4, for small to large adults, respectively.

• A guide to the correct size is determined by comparing the airway length to the vertical distance from the corner of the patient's mouth to the angle of the mandible.

• It is initially inserted 'upside down' as far as the back of the hard palate (Fig. 3.3a), rotated 180° (Fig. 3.3b) and fully inserted until the flange lies in front of the teeth or gums in an edentulous patient (Fig. 3.3c).

NASOPHARYNGEAL AIRWAY

• These are round, malleable plastic tubes, bevelled at the pharyngeal end and flanged at the nasal end.

• They are sized on their internal diameter in millimetres, with length increasing with diameter. The common sizes in adults are 6–8 mm, for small to large adults, respectively.

• A guide to the correct size is made by comparing the diameter to the external nares.

• Prior to insertion, the patency of the nostril (usually the right) should be checked and the airway lubricated.

• The airway is inserted along the floor of the nose, with the bevel facing medially to avoid catching the turbinates (Fig. 3.4).

• A safety pin may be inserted through the flange to prevent inhalation of the airway.

• If obstruction is encountered, force should not be used as severe bleeding may be provoked. Instead, the other nostril can be tried.

PROBLEMS WITH AIRWAYS

The presence of snoring, indrawing of the supraclavicular, suprasternal and intercostal spaces, use of the accessory muscles or paradoxical respiratory movement (see-saw respiration) suggest that the above methods are failing to maintain a patent airway. Common problems arising using these techniques along with a facemask during anaesthesia are:

INSERTION OF AN OROPHARYNGEAL AIRWAY

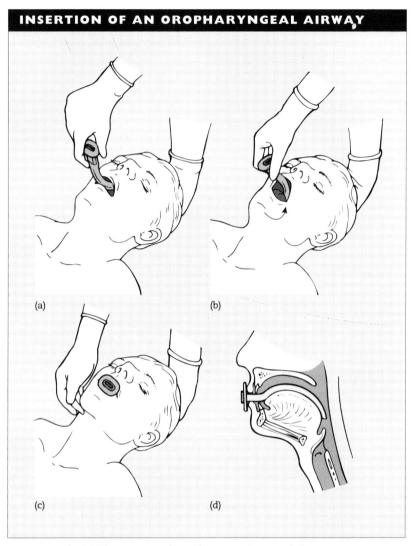

(a)

(b)

(c)

(d)

Fig. 3.3 The sequence of inserting an oropharyngeal airway.

1 inability to maintain a good seal between the patient's face and the mask, particularly in those without teeth;

2 fatigue, when holding the mask for prolonged periods;

3 the risk of aspiration, due to the loss of upper airway reflexes;

4 the anaesthetist is not free to deal with any other problems which may arise.

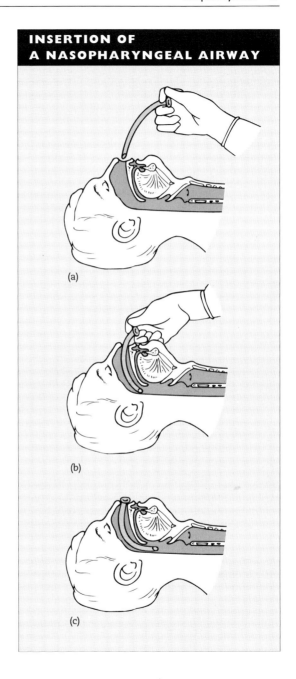

Fig. 3.4 Insertion of a nasopharyngeal airway.

The laryngeal mask airway (LMA) or tracheal intubation may be used to overcome these problems.

The laryngeal mask airway

This device was designed for use in spontaneously breathing patients. It consists of a 'mask' which sits over the laryngeal opening, attached to which is a tube which protrudes from the mouth and connects directly to the anaesthetic breathing system. On the perimeter of the mask is an inflatable cuff which creates a seal and helps to stabilize it. The LMA is produced in a variety of sizes suitable for all patients, from neonates to adults, with sizes 3 and 4 being the most commonly used in female and male adults, respectively. Positive pressure ventilation can be performed via the LMA provided that high inflation pressure is avoided, otherwise leakage occurs past the cuff, reducing ventilation and causing gastric inflation. A version with a reinforced tube is also available. The LMA is reusable, provided that it is sterilized between each patient.

The use of the laryngeal mask overcomes some of the problems of the previous techniques:
• it is not affected by the shape of the patient's face or the absence of teeth;
• the anaesthetist is not required to hold it in position, avoiding fatigue and allowing any other problems to be dealt with;
• it *reduces* the risk of aspiration of regurgitated gastric contents, but does not eliminate it.

Its use is *relatively contraindicated* where there is an increased risk of regurgitation, for example in emergency cases, pregnancy and patients with a hiatus hernia.

Recently, the laryngeal mask has been shown to be useful in two other areas:
1   In difficult tracheal intubation where it will often allow maintenance of the airway. Alternatively, a small diameter tracheal tube or introducer can be passed into the larynx via the LMA.
2   During cardiopulmonary resuscitation, it has been shown that non-anaesthetists are able to insert an LMA more rapidly and successfully than a tracheal tube and achieve more effective ventilation than using a self-inflating bag and facemask. It is likely that in the future the LMA will find a role in airway management during resuscitation.

TECHNIQUE FOR INSERTION

The patient's reflexes must be suppressed to a level similar to that required for the insertion of an oropharyngeal airway to prevent coughing or laryngospasm.

- The cuff is deflated and the mask lightly lubricated (Fig. 3.5a).
- A head tilt is performed, the patient's mouth opened fully and the tip of the mask inserted along the hard palate with the open side facing but not touching the tongue (Fig. 3.5b).
- The mask is then further inserted, using the index finger to provide support for the tube (Fig. 3.5c). Eventually, resistance will be felt at the point where the tip of the mask lies at the upper oesophageal sphincter (Fig. 3.5d).
- The cuff is now fully inflated using an air-filled syringe attached to the valve at the end of the pilot tube (Fig. 3.5e).
- The laryngeal mask is secured either by a length of bandage or adhesive strapping attached to the protruding tube.

Tracheal intubation

This is the best method of providing and securing a clear airway in patients during anaesthesia and resuscitation, but success requires abolition of the laryngeal reflexes. During anaesthesia, this is usually achieved by the administration of a muscle relaxant (see Chapter 4). Deep inhalational anaesthesia or local anaesthesia of the larynx can also be used, but these are usually reserved for use in those patients where difficulty with intubation is anticipated, for example in the presence of airway tumours or immobility of the cervical spine.

COMMON INDICATIONS FOR TRACHEAL INTUBATION

- Where muscle relaxants are used to facilitate surgery (e.g. abdominal and thoracic surgery) thereby necessitating the use of mechanical ventilation.
- In patients with a full stomach, to protect against aspiration of regurgitated gastric contents.
- Where the position of the patient would otherwise make maintenance of the airway difficult, for example the lateral or prone position.
- Where there is competition between surgeon and anaesthetist for the airway (e.g. operations on the head and neck).
- In those patients in whom the airway cannot be satisfactorily maintained by any other technique.
- During cardiopulmonary resuscitation when intubation allows:
    (a) ventilation with 100% oxygen without leaks;
    (b) suction clearance of inhaled debris;
    (c) a route for the administration of drugs.

INSERTION OF A LARYNGEAL MASK AIRWAY

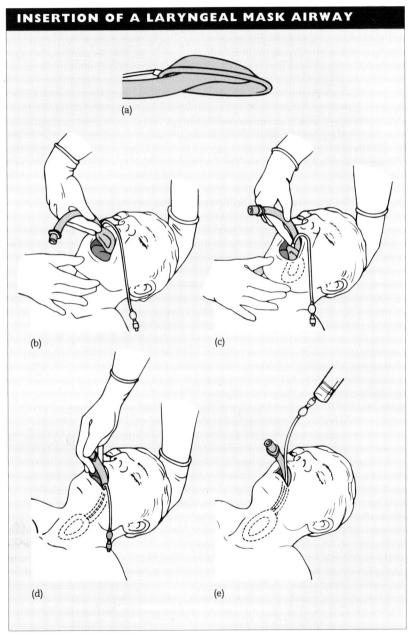

Fig. 3.5 (a–e) Sequence of events in insertion of a laryngeal mask airway (LMA).

EQUIPMENT FOR TRACHEAL INTUBATION

A variety of equipment exists and that chosen will be determined by the circumstances and by the preferences of the individual anaesthetist. The following is a list of the basic needs for *adult oral* intubation.

- *Laryngoscope* with a curved (Macintosh) blade and functioning light.
- *Tracheal tubes* in a variety of sizes and in which the cuffs work. The internal diameter is expressed in millimetres and the length in centimetres. They may be lightly lubricated.
  - (a) For males: 8.0–9.0 mm internal diameter, 22–24 cm length.
  - (b) For females: 7.5–8.5 mm internal diameter, 20–22 cm length.
- *Syringe* to inflate the cuff once the tube is in place.
- *Catheter mount* or 'elbow' to connect the tube to the anaesthetic system or ventilator tubing.
- *Suction*, switched on and immediately to hand in case the patient vomits or regurgitates.
- *Stethoscope* to check correct placement of the tube by listening for breath sounds during ventilation.
- *Extras:* a semi-rigid introducer to help mould the tube to a particular shape; Magill's forceps, designed to reach into the pharynx to remove debris or direct the tip of a tube; bandage or tape to secure the tube.

Tracheal tubes

- These were traditionally manufactured from red rubber and were reusable. However, disposable plastic (PVC) ones are now widely used to eliminate cross-infection and are chemically less irritant to the larynx (Fig. 3.6).
- Tubes are sized according to their internal diameter in millimetres and are manufactured in half-millimetre intervals. They are long enough to be used orally or nasally.
- A standard 15 mm connector is provided to allow connection to the breathing system.
- In adult anaesthesia, a tracheal tube with an inflatable cuff is used to prevent leakage of anaesthetic gases back past the tube when positive pressure ventilation is used. This also helps prevent aspiration of any foreign material into the lungs.
- The cuff is inflated by injecting air from a syringe via a small-diameter tube, at the distal end of which is a one-way valve to prevent deflation and a small pilot balloon which indicates when the cuff is inflated.

A wide variety of specialized tubes have been developed, examples of which are shown in Fig. 3.6.

- Reinforced tubes are used to prevent kinking and subsequent obstruc-

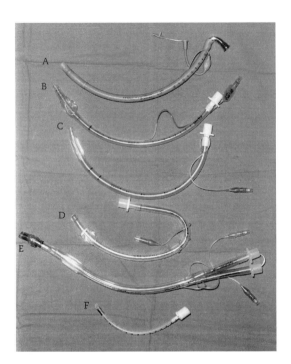

Fig. 3.6 Tracheal tubes: (A) red rubber; (B) PVC; (C) reinforced; (D) preformed (RAE); (E) double lumen; and (F) paediatric (uncuffed).

tion of the tracheal tube as a result of the positioning of the patient's head (Fig. 3.6C).

• Preformed tubes are used during surgery on the head and neck and are designed to take the connections away from the surgical field (Fig. 3.6D).

• Double lumen tubes are effectively two tubes welded together side-by-side, with one tube extending distally beyond the other. They are used during thoracic surgery, and placed such that the distal tube lies within one main bronchus (endobronchial). This allows the other lung to be deflated to facilitate access to, or operation upon, the lung whilst ventilation is maintained via the endobronchial portion (Fig. 3.6E).

• In children under approximately 10 years of age, *uncuffed tubes* are used as a natural seal is provided by the narrowing in the subglottic region (Fig. 3.6F).

THE TECHNIQUE OF ORAL INTUBATION

This requires abolition of the laryngeal reflexes and appropriate monitoring of the patient.

Positioning

The patient is positioned with the neck flexed and the head extended at the atlanto-occipital joint. This is the so-called 'sniffing the morning air' position. The patient's mouth is fully opened using the index finger and thumb of the *right* hand in a scissor action.

Laryngoscopy

The laryngoscope is always held in the *left* hand and the blade is introduced into the mouth along the right-hand side of the tongue, displacing it to the left. The blade is advanced until the tip lies in the gap between the base of the tongue and the epiglottis, the vallecula. Force is then applied *in the direction in which the handle of the laryngoscope is pointing*, the effort coming from the upper arm not the wrist, to lift the tongue and epiglottis to expose the larynx. This should be seen as a triangular opening, with the apex anteriorly and the whitish coloured true cords laterally (Fig. 3.7).

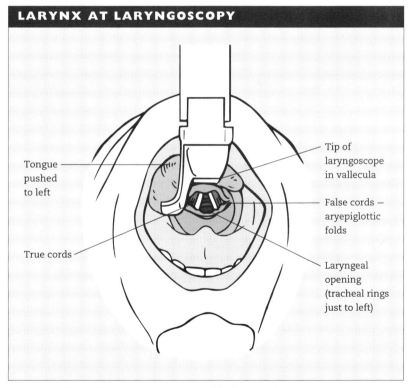

LARYNX AT LARYNGOSCOPY

Tongue pushed to left

Tip of laryngoscope in vallecula

False cords – aryepiglottic folds

True cords

Laryngeal opening (tracheal rings just to left)

Fig. 3.7 Diagram showing a view of the larynx at laryngoscopy.

Intubation

The tracheal tube is introduced into the right side of the mouth, advanced and *seen to pass through the cords* until the cuff lies just below the cords. The tube is then held firmly by the fingers of the right hand and the laryngoscope is carefully removed. The cuff is then inflated sufficiently to prevent any leak during ventilation. Finally the position of the tube is confirmed by listening for breath sounds in both axillae and it is then secured in place.

For nasotracheal intubation; a well-lubricated tube is introduced usually via the right nostril along the floor of the nose with the bevel pointing medially to avoid damage to the turbinates. It is advanced into the oropharynx, where it is usually visualized using a laryngoscope in the manner described above. It can then either be advanced directly into the larynx by pushing on the proximal end, or the tip picked up with Magill's forceps (which are designed not to impair the view of the larynx) and directed into the larynx. The procedure then continues as for oral intubation.

DIFFICULT INTUBATION

Occasionally, intubation of the trachea is made difficult because of an inability to visualize the larynx. This may have been predicted at the preoperative assessment or may be unexpected. A variety of techniques have been described to help solve this problem and include the following:

• manipulation of the thyroid cartilage by downwards and upwards pressure by an assistant to try and bring the larynx or its posterior aspect into view;

• at laryngoscopy, a gum elastic bougie, 60 cm long, is inserted into the trachea, over which the tracheal tube is 'railroaded' into place;

• a fibreoptic bronchoscope is introduced into the trachea via the mouth or nose and is used as a guide over which a tube can be passed into the trachea. This technique has the advantage that it can be used in either anaesthetized or awake patients.

COMPLICATIONS OF TRACHEAL INTUBATION

The following is one method of categorizing them, but it is not an attempt to cover all occurrences.

Hypoxia

• *Oesophageal intubation.* This is best detected by measuring the carbon dioxide in expired gas; less than 0.2% indicates oesophageal intubation. An alternative is to attach a 50 ml 'bladder' syringe to the tracheal tube and withdraw the plunger rapidly (Wee's oesophageal detector). If the tracheal tube is in the oesophagus, resistance is felt and air cannot be aspirated; if it is in the trachea, air is easily aspirated. Less reliable signs are 'burping' sounds as gas escapes, diminished breath sounds on auscultation, decreased chest movement on ventilation and gurgling sounds over the epigastrium. Pulse oximetry only changes late, particularly if the patient has been preoxygenated.

NB. If there is any doubt about the position of the tube then it should be removed and the patient ventilated via a facemask.

• *Failed intubation and inability to ventilate the patient.* This is usually a result of abnormal anatomy or airway pathology. Many cases are predictable at the preoperative assessment (see page 6).

• *Failed ventilation after intubation.* Possible causes include the tube becoming kinked, disconnected, or inserted too far and passing into one main bronchus, severe bronchospasm and tension pneumothorax.

• *Aspiration.* Regurgitated gastric contents can cause blockage of the airways directly or secondary to laryngeal spasm and bronchospasm. Cricoid pressure can be used to reduce the risk of regurgitation prior to intubation (see below).

Trauma

• Directly during laryngoscopy and insertion of the tube to lips, teeth, tongue, pharynx, larynx, trachea, and nose and nasopharynx during nasal intubation; causing soft tissue swelling or bleeding.

• Indirectly to the mandible (dislocation), and the cervical spine and cord, particularly where there is pre-existing degenerative disease or trauma.

Reflex activity

• *Hypertension and dysrhythmias.* This occurs in response to intubation and may jeopardize patients with coronary artery disease, aortic or intracranial aneurysms. In patients at risk, specific action is taken to attenuate the response, for example pretreatment with β-blockers, potent analgesics (fentanyl, alfentanil) or intravenous lignocaine.

• *Vomiting.* This may be stimulated when laryngoscopy is attempted in patients who are inadequately anaesthetized. It is more frequent when there is material in the stomach; for example in emergencies when the patient is not starved, in patients with intestinal obstruction, or when gastric emptying is delayed, as after opiate analgesics or following trauma.

• *Laryngeal spasm.* Reflex adduction of the vocal cords as a result of stimulation of the epiglottis or larynx.

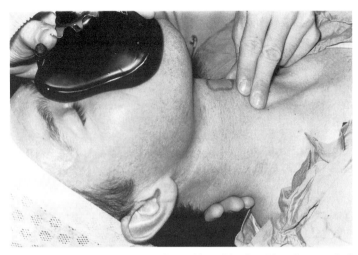

Fig. 3.8 Sellick's manoeuvre. Note the position of the thyroid cartilage marked on the patient's neck.

CRICOID PRESSURE (SELLICK'S MANOEUVRE)

The cricoid cartilage is the only complete ring of cartilage in the larynx. Pressure exerted upon it anteroposteriorly forces the whole ring posteriorly, compressing the oesophagus against the body of the sixth cervical vertebra, thereby preventing passive regurgitation. It is performed by an assistant using the thumb and first two fingers to apply the pressure whilst the other hand is placed behind the patient's neck to stabilize it (Fig. 3.8). Pressure is applied as the patient loses consciousness and maintained until the tube has been successfully inserted, the cuff inflated and tube position confirmed. If the patient starts to actively vomit, pressure should be released due to the risk of the oesophagus rupturing, and the patient should be turned onto their side to minimize aspiration.

Emergency airway techniques

These must only be used when *all other techniques have failed* to secure and maintain an airway and oxygenation in either an anaesthetized patient or one undergoing resuscitation.

▌ *Needle cricothyroidotomy.* The cricothyroid membrane is identified and punctured using a large bore cannula (12–14 gauge) attached to a syringe. Aspiration of air confirms that the cannula lies within the trachea. The cannula is then angled to about 45° caudally and advanced off the needle into the trachea (Fig. 3.9). A high-flow oxygen supply is then attached to

NEEDLE CRICOTHYROIDOTOMY AND EQUIPMENT FOR OXYGEN DELIVERY

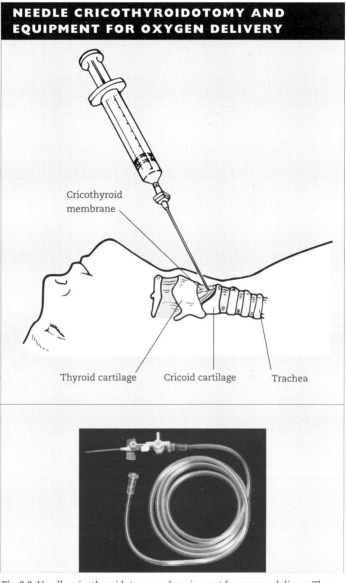

Cricothyroid membrane

Thyroid cartilage   Cricoid cartilage   Trachea

Fig. 3.9 Needle cricothyroidotomy and equipment for oxygen delivery. The three-way tap is set with all ports open. Occluding the open port diverts oxygen to the patient. Luer-locks on the cannula, three-way tap and tubing prevent disconnection by the pressures generated.

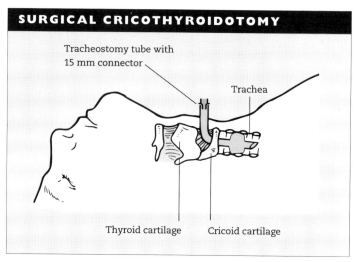

Fig. 3.10 Surgical cricothyroidotomy.

the cannula and insufflated for 1 second followed by a 4-second rest. Expiration occurs via the upper airway as normal. This technique only oxygenates the patient and does not eliminate carbon dioxide. It is therefore limited to about 30 minutes use while a definitive airway is created.

2 *Surgical cricothyroidotomy.* This involves making an incision through the cricothyroid membrane to allow the introduction of a 5.0–6.0 mm diameter tracheostomy tube or tracheal tube (Fig. 3.10). It is more difficult to perform, and results in significantly more bleeding, than the above. The advantages are that once a tube of this diameter has been inserted, the patient can be adequately ventilated, ensuring oxygenation, elimination of carbon dioxide and the airway suctioned to remove any blood or debris.

Further reading

Aitkinson RS, Rushman GB, Lee JA. *A Synopsis of Anaesthesia*, 10th edn. Bristol: Wright, 1987.

Beunmof JL. Management of the difficult adult airway. *Anesthesiology* 1991; **75**: 1087–110.

Driscoll PA, Gwinnutt CL, Jimmerson CL, Goodall O (eds). *Trauma Resuscitation: The Team Approach.* London: Macmillan Press Ltd, 1993.

O'Meara ME, Jones JG. The laryngeal mask. *British Medical Journal* 1993; **306**: 224–5.

CHAPTER 4

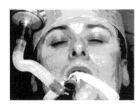

Drugs Associated with Anaesthesia

The anaesthetist has to be familiar with a wide range of drugs to facilitate the safe and effective conduct of anaesthesia. Unlike most other branches of medicine, these are almost always administered parenterally; either intravenously or via inhalation. Unfortunately, as well as their desired effect on the central nervous system, these drugs have undesirable actions on many other body systems of which the anaesthetist must be fully aware.

Intravenous anaesthetic (induction) agents

These are drugs which are used to start (induce) anaesthesia. After intravenous (i.v.) administration, consciousness is lost in little more than the time it takes for these drugs to get from the site of administration to the brain (one arm–brain circulation time). Generally, consciousness is regained by redistribution from the brain to other tissues. Currently, only propofol is also used to maintain anaesthesia. Anaesthesia can also be induced by the inhalation of an increasing concentration of a volatile agent.

Because of the adverse effects of the i.v. agents on the cardiovascular system, much lower doses should be administered in elderly, frail or shocked patients.

SODIUM THIOPENTONE (INTRAVAL)

This is a short-acting barbiturate, the dose required for induction is usually between 2 and 7 mg/kg. Induction of anaesthesia is rapid and smooth, taking about 15–20 seconds, except in those whose circulation is delayed, for example patients who are elderly, hypovolaemic, or have cardiac disease. Patients may comment on being able to taste onions or garlic during administration. Consciousness usually returns after 4–10 minutes as the result of redistribution, followed by a prolonged period ($\approx$ 24 hours) of metabolism by the liver and excretion by the kidneys. Repeated doses are associated with accumulation and delayed recovery.

Systemic effects

- Hypotension occurs secondary to myocardial depression and venodilatation. This is exaggerated in those who are hypovolaemic or have a limited cardiovascular reserve.
- A short period of breath holding occurs followed by depression of ventilation.
- Sodium thiopentone is a potent anticonvulsant. Cerebral metabolism, blood flow and intracranial pressure are reduced.
- As with all barbiturates, administration may exacerbate porphyria.

PROPOFOL (DIPRIVAN)

Propofol is prepared as an emulsion. The dose required to induce anaesthesia is usually between 1.5 and 2.5 mg/kg. Thirty to forty per cent of patients complain of pain or burning on injection. Induction of anaesthesia is rapid but less definite than with thiopentone. Involuntary movements are sometimes seen. After 4–7 minutes, there is a rapid, full recovery of consciousness, a property which has made propofol popular for day-case surgery. Postoperative nausea and vomiting are uncommon. A constant infusion (or repeated bolus doses) can be used to maintain anaesthesia.

Systemic effects

- Hypotension is common, secondary to vasodilatation.
- Apnoea is common after an induction dose and may last for 40–50 seconds.
- Ventilation and the response to carbon dioxide are depressed. Laryngeal reflexes appear to be depressed, laryngeal spasm is uncommon.
- Cerebral metabolism and blood flow are reduced along with intracranial pressure.
- Muscle relaxation is more pronounced after propofol, particularly when used as a constant infusion to maintain anaesthesia.

ETOMIDATE (HYPNOMIDATE)

The dose for induction of anaesthesia is 0.2–0.3 mg/kg. Pain on injection is common. Induction is rapid, but is frequently associated with muscle twitching and involuntary movement. Recovery occurs after 4–8 minutes, following redistribution from the brain. Etomidate is non-cumulative, even after several doses.

Systemic effects

- Causes a slight fall in cardiac output and minimal vasodilatation. Blood pressure is better maintained than with other agents, making it popular for use in sick patients.
- Causes dose-dependent depression of ventilation and a decreased ventilatory response to carbon dioxide.
- Reduces cerebral metabolism, blood flow and intracranial pressure, and it is anticonvulsant.
- It does not cause histamine release and allergic reactions are extremely rare.
- Despite being non-cumulative, prolonged use suppresses adrenocortical function, impairing recovery in critically ill patients.

KETAMINE (KETALAR)

The i.v. dose is 1–2 mg/kg, following which consciousness is lost over 1 minute, lasting for 10–20 minutes. Ketamine can also be administered intramuscularly to induce anaesthesia. The intramuscular (i.m.) dose is 5–10 mg/kg and it may take 8–10 minutes to lose consciousness. The subsequent duration of action is variable. Repeat boluses or an infusion can be administered to maintain anaesthesia. Vivid hallucinations are common during recovery and can be minimized by the concurrent use of a benzodiazepine (e.g. midazolam).

Systemic effects

- Heart rate, blood pressure and cardiac output are well maintained even in shocked patients, making it useful during emergency surgery.
- There is minimal depression of ventilation.
- Laryngeal reflexes are also maintained better than with other agents and bronchodilatation occurs.

Advantages

The ability to administer ketamine by i.m. injection is useful when venous access is difficult. The profound analgesic effects can be obtained at sub-anaesthetic doses. This property is utilized when patients, often children, undergo repeated minor painful procedures, for example burns dressings. It is occasionally used as the sole agent in adverse circumstances, for example in prehospital care to facilitate extrication of severely injured victims.

METHOHEXITONE (BRIETAL)

This is a shorter acting barbiturate than thiopentone. It was originally popular for short procedures and day cases because of the improved recovery compared with thiopentone. It has now largely been superseded by propofol.

MIDAZOLAM

This is a short-acting, water-soluble benzodiazepine. It is not a true induction agent as it does not produce a rapid loss of consciousness. The dose required to induce anaesthesia is between 0.1 and 0.3 mg/kg. It may take 30–45 seconds before consciousness is lost with the end-point being very indistinct. Recovery occurs after 10–15 minutes and is associated with a longer period of amnesia.

Systemic effects

- Causes relatively little cardiovascular depression.
- It is a potent respiratory depressant, particularly in the elderly.
- It has mild anticonvulsant and muscle relaxant properties.

Inhalational induction

This may be used when i.v. induction of anaesthesia is not practical, for example in an uncooperative child or a patient with a lack of suitable veins. Anaesthesia is induced relatively slowly and respiration is preserved. This is therefore a useful technique in patients with airway compromise, when an i.v. agent may cause apnoea, and ventilation and oxygenation become impossible with catastrophic results.

The patient breathes an increasing concentration of an inhalational agent in oxygen (if there is airway compromise), or in a mixture of oxygen and nitrous oxide. Adequacy of anaesthesia is assessed (and overdosage avoided) based on clinical signs or 'stages of anaesthesia'. The original description of these stages by A.E. Guedel was based on using ether, but the main features can still be seen using modern agents. However, they will be modified by the concurrent administration of opiates or anticholinergics.

First stage

This lasts from starting the inhalation until consciousness is lost. The pupils will be normal in size and reactive, muscle tone is normal and breathing uses intercostal muscles and the diaphragm.

Second stage

In this period there may be breath-holding, struggling and coughing. It is often referred to as the stage of excitation. The pupils will be dilated and there is loss of the eyelash reflex.

Third stage

This is the stage of surgical anaesthesia. It is classically subdivided into four further planes. There is reduction in respiratory activity, with progressive intercostal paralysis. Muscle tone is also reduced and laryngeal reflexes lost. The pupils start by being slightly constricted and gradually dilate. This stage ends with diaphragmatic paralysis.

Fourth stage

This constitutes an anaesthetic catastrophe, with apnoea, loss of all reflex activity and fixed dilated pupils.

Clearly, the depth of anaesthesia achieved will depend upon whether surgery is to be performed with the patient still breathing spontaneously, or whether induction is to be followed by a balanced technique with muscle relaxants, intubation and controlled ventilation. As well as the observations listed above, the anaesthetic agent will have effects on all of the other body systems, which will need appropriate monitoring. Further details of the specific effects of the various agents used are given below.

Inhalational agents and intravenous infusions

Following induction, anaesthesia is most often maintained by the administration of nitrous oxide plus an anaesthetic vapour in oxygen. The concentration of the vapour (and nitrous oxide) administered to maintain anaesthesia is expressed as the percentage by volume. In order to compare the efficacy of anaesthetic agents and their potential side-effects on other systems, the concept of MAC is used, rather than simply comparing a fixed inspired concentration. MAC is a measure of the minimum alveolar concentration of an inhalational agent that has to be achieved to prevent movement in 50% of subjects following a surgical stimulus. A higher alveolar concentration will need to be achieved for agents that have a low potency (e.g. desflurane) compared with those that have a high potency (e.g. halothane). Nevertheless at 1 MAC, or multiples thereof, the anaesthetic effect will be the same and a comparison of the side-effects can be made.

The anaesthetic effects of the inhalational agents are additive and therefore two values of MAC are often quoted—the value in oxygen and the value when administered with a stated percentage of nitrous oxide, which will clearly be less (Table 4.1).

An alternative method of expressing the potency of inhalational agents is as the alveolar concentration which prevents movement in response to

COMPARISON OF MAC VALUES

	Halothane (%)	Enflurane (%)	Isoflurane (%)	Desflurane (%)	Sevoflurane (%)
In 100% oxygen	0.75	1.58	1.28	6	2.2
In 70% nitrous oxide	0.29	0.57	0.56	2.8	1.2

Table 4.1 Comparison of minimum alveolar concentration (MAC) values for the currently used agents.

surgery in 95% of patients—the AD95. This gives values approximately 1.5 times the MAC value and is probably a more relevant figure for clinical anaesthesia.

The value of MAC is dependent upon various other factors. It is reduced by increasing age, hypotension, hypothermia, hypothyroidism and concurrent use of opioids. It is increased in infants, patients with a pyrexia, and in those who are chronic drug abusers.

NITROUS OXIDE (N_2O)

Nitrous oxide is a colourless, sweet-smelling, non-irritant gas. It is a good analgesic but a poor anaesthetic. The maximum safe concentration that can be administered (without the risk of hypoxia) is approximately 70%, which does not guarantee unconsciousness or anaesthesia sufficient to allow surgery to proceed. At the end of anaesthesia, rapid excretion of nitrous oxide into the alveoli dilutes any oxygen present (diffusion hypoxia or 'Fink effect'). If the patient is breathing air then significant hypoxia can occur. This can be overcome by increasing the inspired oxygen concentration during recovery.

Nitrous oxide is premixed with oxygen as a 50:50 mixture called 'Entonox' which is used as an analgesic in obstetrics and by the emergency services.

Systemic effects

• Has little effect on cardiac output or blood pressure unless patient has severe cardiac disease.

• Causes a slight increase in the respiratory rate and a decrease in the tidal volume. It decreases the ventilatory response to carbon dioxide and hypoxia.

• It diffuses more rapidly into air-filled cavities than any nitrogen can escape, causing either a rise in pressure (e.g. in the middle ear) or an increase in volume (e.g. within the gut or of an air embolus).

- May cause bone-marrow suppression by inhibiting the production of factors necessary for the synthesis of DNA. The length of exposure necessary may be as short as a few hours, and recovery usually occurs within 1 week.

HALOTHANE (FLUOTHANE)

This is a colourless, volatile liquid with a pleasant odour. It is relatively non-irritant to the respiratory tract. Induction of anaesthesia can be achieved with 2–4% and maintenance with 0.5–1.5% inspired concentration when administered with 70% nitrous oxide and 30% oxygen. It has no analgesic action and is most commonly used with nitrous oxide and oxygen in spontaneously breathing patients or as part of a balanced technique. It can be used with soda lime in a circle system (see page 29).

Systemic effects

- Halothane causes a dose-related fall in blood pressure as a result of myocardial depression and vasodilation.
- Dysrhythmias are common and include sinus bradycardias and nodal rhythm. The myocardium is sensitized to circulating levels of adrenaline, both endogenous (light anaesthesia) and exogenous (infiltration) causing ventricular extrasystoles and bigeminy.
- Causes depression of ventilation and the ventilatory response to both hypercarbia and hypoxia is lost.
- There is slight bronchial dilatation and both pharyngeal and laryngeal protective reflexes are depressed. Non-irritant to the respiratory tract.
- Increases cerebral blood flow and the intracranial pressure.
- Relaxation of skeletal and smooth muscle, including the pregnant uterus, which may increase blood loss during Caesarian section.
- Significant amounts of halothane are metabolized in the liver ($\approx 20\%$) and excreted over many days.

Disadvantages

The main disadvantages are that it can trigger malignant hyperpyrexia (see page 69) and has been implicated as a cause of hepatotoxicity 'halothane hepatitis' (see below).

Halothane hepatitis

The precise link between the use of halothane and the subsequent development of hepatitis remains unclear. The incidence is extremely low, being in the region of 1 : 10 000–20 000 halothane administrations. The clinical picture is one of jaundice with a massive rise in plasma aminotransferases several days after the exposure to halothane, associated with severe hepatic necrosis. The mortality rate is approximately 50%. There are two current theories of causation: (i) the production of a hepatotoxic metabolite in the presence of hypoxia; and (ii) the production of a metabolite which can bind to liver proteins acting as an antigen.

The current recommendations for the use of halothane in clinical practice are as follows:

• Severe liver damage is unlikely to occur after a single exposure in adults.

• Repeat administration to adults, often over an interval of less than 3 months should be avoided, particularly in obese, middle-aged females.

• The risk to children appears to be much less and they can receive repeat administrations.

• If a repeat administration is necessary in an adult, every effort should be made to ensure that the previous exposure was uneventful. If this is the case, the reasons for repeating halothane should be documented. If problems are identified, halothane must not be repeated.

• Liver disease itself is not a contraindication to the use of halothane (providing that it was not halothane-induced!).

ENFLURANE (ETHRANE)

Enflurane is a colourless liquid, with a pungent smell. It is slightly more irritant than halothane. It is less potent than halothane, with 1.5–2% needed for maintenance of anaesthesia when used with 70% nitrous oxide and 30% oxygen. Induction, recovery and changes in depth of anaesthesia can be achieved relatively quickly, although the former is limited by its pungency.

Systemic effects

• Enflurane causes a dose-dependent fall in blood pressure and ventilation.

• The heart rate is well maintained and the cardiac rhythm is stable, even in the presence of raised levels of catecholamines, making it safer for use when adrenaline-containing solutions (usually local anaesthetics) are also being administered.

• Increases cerebral blood flow and at high concentrations (> 3%) causes an abnormal increase in electroencephalogram (EEG) activity. Not recommended for use in patients known to suffer from, or who are prone to, epilepsy.

• Similar effects to halothane on skeletal and smooth muscle, including the uterus.

• Small amounts are metabolized in the liver (< 2%), which may contribute to the very low incidence of hepatitis even after repeat exposure.

- Malignant hyperpyrexia may be triggered, but at a lower incidence than following halothane.

ISOFLURANE (FORANE)

This is a colourless liquid with a very pungent smell. It is mildly irritant to breathe which limits its use for inhalation induction. Isoflurane lies between halothane and enflurane in its potency; up to 5% is required for induction and 1–1.5% for maintenance of anaesthesia when used with 70% nitrous oxide and 30% oxygen. It is associated with a rapid recovery from anaesthesia with minimal hangover effects, making it popular for use in day-case surgery. Currently, isoflurane is the inhalational agent of choice for neurosurgical anaesthesia because of its minimal effect on cerebral blood flow and intracranial pressure.

Systemic effects

- Isoflurane causes a dose-dependent fall in blood pressure due mainly to peripheral vasodilatation.
- The pulse rate is maintained, with a tendency to tachycardia in young patients due to maintenance of the baroreceptor reflexes. Cardiac rhythm is stable, even in the presence of high levels of catecholamines.
- Ventilation is depressed with tidal volume affected more than respiratory rate and the ventilatory response to hypoxia and hypercarbia is also reduced.
- It has minimal effect on cerebral blood flow and intracranial pressure at low concentrations (< 1 MAC).
- Isoflurane provides good relaxation of skeletal muscle, potentiating the effects of non-depolarizing muscle relaxants and causes relaxation of uterine muscles.
- Hepatic and renal blood flow are well maintained with metabolism of very small amounts (<0.2%). This minimizes the risk of inducing hepatitis.

DESFLURANE (SUPRANE)

This is one of the two most recently introduced volatile agents but is very irritant to breathe. It has a boiling point of only 23°C which makes administration technically more complex. Desflurane is a weak anaesthetic agent, compensated for by the fact that it has the lowest solubility of all the current agents (see below), allowing a more rapid induction, change in depth of anaesthesia and recovery than with the other inhalational agents.

Systemic effects

- At low concentrations vasodilatation may cause the blood pressure to

fall, but at higher concentrations (2 MAC) cardiac performance may actually be increased. There is no effect on heart rhythm.
• Ventilatory depression occurs with a reduction in tidal volume, a slight increase in respiratory rate and a reduction in the ventilatory response to carbon dioxide.
• It has similar effects on cerebral blood flow and intracranial pressure as isoflurane.
• As a result of the molecules' stability, it undergoes virtually no metabolism and is unlikely to have any adverse hepatic or renal effects.

SEVOFLURANE

This is the second recent inhalational agent introduced, and is a colourless liquid which is non-irritant to the respiratory tract. It is a relatively weak anaesthetic agent, but like desflurane this is compensated for by its low solubility which facilitates induction, changes in depth and recovery from anaesthesia. Ease of inhalation and its insolubility make sevoflurane attractive for use in short cases, for example anaesthesia for day-case surgery where speed and quality of recovery is important, and for inhalational induction.

Systemic effects

• Sevoflurane decreases the blood pressure in a dose-related manner, primarily due to peripheral vasodilatation.
• There is relatively little effect on heart rate and cardiac rhythm remains stable. Ventilatory depression occurs with a decrease in the ventilatory response to carbon dioxide.
• The effects on cerebral blood flow are similar to those for isoflurane.

ETHER (DIETHYL ETHER)

This was the first agent to successfully produce surgical anaesthesia. The increasing use of electrical apparatus in the modern operating theatre, combined with the flammability of ether over a wide range of concentrations, predispose to an unacceptable risk of fires and explosions and its main use nowadays is in developing countries which lack such equipment. Ether is a moderately potent anaesthetic agent (MAC ≈ 2%), however, induction and recovery are slow because it is extremely soluble.

THE SOLUBILITY OF
INHALATIONAL ANAESTHETIC AGENTS

Inhalational anaesthetics, like the i.v. anaesthetics, exert their effect on the central nervous system. Diffusion of anaesthetic from the alveoli into the blood and delivery to the brain occurs with remarkable speed and the partial pressure in the brain (responsible for the anaesthetic effect) follows that in the alveoli very closely. Consequently, the rate at which the alveolar partial pressure can be changed determines the rate of change in brain partial pressure and hence speed of induction, change in depth and recovery from anaesthesia.

One of the main determinants of alveolar partial pressure is the solubility of the inhalational anaesthetic agent in blood (or more precisely its blood : gas partition coefficient). If an agent is very *insoluble* (e.g. desflurane), then on administration, little is removed from the alveoli by the pulmonary blood. The alveolar partial pressure (and brain partial pressure) rise quickly and anaesthesia is rapidly induced. Changes in the inspired concentration are reflected in the alveolar partial pressure, allowing depth of anaesthesia to be adjusted with equal speed. In contrast, if a *soluble* agent (e.g. ether) is administered, large amounts diffuse from the alveoli into the pulmonary blood, limiting the rate of rise of alveolar and hence brain partial pressure. Consequently, induction will be slower as will be any subsequent attempts to adjust the depth of anaesthesia.

Recovery from anaesthesia follows similar principles in reverse. Only a small amount of an insoluble agent will have to be excreted to allow brain partial pressure to fall. With a more soluble agent, a larger amount will need to be excreted, which will take proportionately longer.

Other factors which determine the speed at which the alveolar concentration will rise include the following:
• The inspired concentration—clinically the pungency or irritation of the inhalational agents limits the use of high concentrations.
• Alveolar ventilation—this is most pronounced for agents with a high solubility. As large amounts are removed from the alveoli, increasing ventilation ensures more rapid replacement.
• An increased cardiac output results in a greater pulmonary blood flow, increasing uptake thereby lowering the alveolar partial pressure. A low cardiac output will result in a reduced peripheral blood flow, and blood returning to the lungs will still contain some anaesthetic. The partial pressure gradient between alveoli and blood is reduced, the net result being that the alveolar concentration rises more rapidly.

PROPOFOL (2,6-DIISOPROPYLPHENOL)

In order to use an i.v. anaesthetic agent to maintain anaesthesia, it must be rapidly eliminated or metabolized to inactive substances in order to prevent accumulation and delay recovery. Currently, propofol is the best agent for this technique; ketamine is associated with an unpleasant recovery, etomidate suppresses steroid synthesis and recovery after barbiturates is prolonged due to their accumulation. Propofol can be administered either as repeat boluses or as a constant infusion.

As with the inhalational agents, a minimum concentration of an i.v. agent is required in the brain to maintain anaesthesia. This is initially achieved by giving *an i.v. bolus or a very rapid infusion*. This is then followed by a constant infusion at a lower rate to maintain the blood concentration. When only i.v. agents are used to induce and maintain anaesthesia, the term 'total intravenous anaesthesia' (TIVA) is often used.

Advantages of total intravenous anaesthesia

- Risks such as malignant hyperpyrexia, hepatitis and the problems associated with nitrous oxide can be avoided.
- It is useful in neurosurgical anaesthesia as cerebral blood flow and intracranial pressure are reduced.
- Fewer drugs are used, thereby reducing the risks of adverse reactions and interactions.
- Pollution is reduced.
- Advocates of this technique claim a better quality of recovery.

However, accurate devices are required to deliver constant infusions (e.g. electronic syringe pumps), a situation analogous to the vaporizers required for inhalational agents.

Neuromuscular blocking drugs and their antagonism

Prior to the introduction of neuromuscular blocking drugs, muscle relaxation to facilitate surgical access was achieved either by using high concentrations of inhalational anaesthetic agents or by regional anaesthesia. The introduction of curare (tubocurarine) in 1942 changed this, allowing muscle relaxation to be achieved whilst less anaesthetic was administered.

Neuromuscular blocking drugs work by interfering with the normal action of acetylcholine, blocking the receptors on the postsynaptic muscle membrane (and possibly other sites). Muscle relaxants are divided into two groups, the names of which are thought to reflect their mode of action.

DEPOLARIZING MUSCLE RELAXANTS

Only suxamethonium is in regular clinical use. Following administration it 'mimics' the action of acetylcholine at the receptors on the motor end plate, resulting in depolarization of the muscle membrane. This is seen as uncoordinated muscle contractions (fasciculations). Unlike acetylcholine, suxamethonium is not metabolized by acetylcholinesterase and the depolarization persists for several minutes, preventing further muscle activity. Ultimately, hydrolysis by plasma (pseudo-)cholinesterase occurs, with restoration of normal neuromuscular transmission.

Suxamethonium

This is used almost exclusively intravenously (but can be administered intramuscularly or subcutaneously) to ensure rapid, predictable and profound relaxation. The dose in adults is 1.5 mg/kg. Muscle fasciculations are followed by profound relaxation in 40–60 seconds, lasting 4–6 minutes. The rapid onset makes it the drug of choice to facilitate tracheal intubation in patients likely to regurgitate and aspirate.

Systemic effects

• No direct effect on the cardiovascular, respiratory or central nervous systems. Bradycardia secondary to vagal stimulation is common after very large or repeated doses, necessitating pretreatment with atropine.
• A massive rise in serum K^+ may provoke dysrhythmias in certain patients:
    (a) in burns patients, maximal 3 weeks to 3 months after the burn;
    (b) in denervation injury, for example spinal cord trauma, maximal after 1 week;
    (c) muscle dystrophies, for example Duchenne's;
    (d) after crush injury.
• Administration of suxamethonium is associated with:
    (a) malignant hyperpyrexia in susceptible patients (see below);
    (b) increased intraocular pressure which may cause loss of vitreous in penetrating eye injuries;
    (c) muscular pain around the limb girdles, most common 24 hours after administration in young adults;
    (d) histamine release — suxamethonium is the commonest relaxant implicated in anaphylactoid reactions;
    (e) prolonged apnoea in patients with pseudocholinesterase deficiency.

Pseudocholinesterase deficiency

A variety of genes have been identified which are involved in pseudocholinesterase production. The most significant resulting genotypes are:
• normal homozygotes with sufficient enzyme to hydrolyse suxamethonium in 4–6 minutes (950 per 1000 population);
• atypical heterozygotes with slightly reduced enzyme levels — suxamethonium lasts 10–20 minutes (50 per 1000);

- atypical homozygotes with marked deficiency of enzyme—members of this group are apnoeic for up to 2 hours after suxamethonium (< 1 per 1000).

Treatment of the third group consists of ventilatory support with maintenance of anaesthesia or sedation until recovery occurs. The patient should subsequently be warned and given a card carrying details and, because of its inherited nature, the remainder of the family should be investigated appropriately.

NON-DEPOLARIZING MUSCLE RELAXANTS

These drugs compete with acetylcholine and block its access to the post-synaptic receptor sites on the muscle but do not cause depolarization and are sometimes referred to as competitive relaxants. (They may also block prejunctional receptors responsible for facilitating the release of acetylcholine.) They are administered intravenously and the time to onset of maximum effect is relatively slow compared with suxamethonium, but it is generally 1.5–3 minutes. Duration of action is 15–45 minutes, depending upon the choice of drug and the dose used. Non-depolarizing relaxants are used in two ways:

1   following suxamethonium to maintain relaxation during surgery;
2   to facilitate tracheal intubation in non-urgent situations.

Although recovery of normal neuromuscular function eventually occurs spontaneously after the use of these drugs, it is usually accelerated by the administration of an anticholinesterase (see below).

Atracurium (Tracrium)

An initial dose of 0.5 mg/kg produces relaxation, allowing intubation after 90–120 seconds and this lasts for 20–25 minutes. During prolonged procedures, the administration of an infusion or intermittent increments can be used to maintain relaxation. At body temperature and pH, atracurium undergoes spontaneous degradation via a process called 'Hofmann elimination' and is therefore stored at 4°C to reduce the rate of spontaneous degradation. It is the relaxant of choice in patients with either renal or hepatic dysfunction. Its actions will be prolonged in hypothermic patients, for example during cardiac surgery. It may cause histamine release but this is usually limited to cutaneous manifestations.

Vecuronium (Norcuron)

An initial dose of 0.1 mg/kg produces relaxation in 90–120 seconds, lasting for 15–20 minutes. This can be extended by increasing the dose to 0.15–0.2 mg/kg. For longer procedures it is more common to use an infusion. Vecuronium does not cause histamine release. Small amounts of vecuronium are metabolized by the liver, but mainly it is excreted unchanged in the bile.

Mivacurium (Mivacron)

Structurally, Mivacurium is related to atracurium. It is regarded as a short-acting, non-depolarizing relaxant. The initial dose is 0.15 mg/kg and this provides relaxation allowing intubation in 2 minutes. The duration of action is only 10–15 minutes, after which time recovery is sufficiently rapid not to need the routine administration of an anticholinesterase. The main advantage of mivacurium is in day-case surgery or short surgical procedures where muscle relaxation is required, allowing suxamethonium to be avoided.

Rocuronium (Esmeron)

This is an intermediate duration relaxant. Following an initial dose of 0.6 mg/kg, relaxation is achieved in around 60 seconds (i.e. approaching that for suxamethonium) and maintained for a period of 20–30 minutes. Rocuronium is useful in those patients in whom rapid intubation is required but there is a need to avoid the use of suxamethonium.

Tubocurarine, curare (Jexin)

This was the first non-depolarizing relaxant to be used in clinical practice. It is often referred to as a long-acting relaxant. Tubocurarine is obtained from the plant *Chondodendron tomentosum* which grows in the Amazon, and is traditionally used by the local Indians as an arrow poison.

The initial dose is 0.5 mg/kg which takes approximately 3 minutes to provide sufficient relaxation to allow intubation and provides adequate relaxation for surgery for 30–40 minutes.

Tubocurarine causes hypotension secondary to ganglion block and vasodilatation, a property used to reduce surgical bleeding, for example during middle ear surgery. It releases histamine, which may contribute to the fall in blood pressure. It is not metabolized and is excreted mainly in the urine (70%).

Pancuronium (Pavulon)

The initial dose of pancuronium is 0.1 mg/kg, which allows intubation in about 2 minutes and relaxation lasts about 30–40 minutes. Pulse rate and blood pressure are both elevated after the use of pancuronium, an effect mediated by blocking noradrenaline uptake. Histamine release is very rare and hence it is useful in patients with asthma.

ASSESSMENT OF NEUROMUSCULAR BLOCKADE

Clinical assessment requires a conscious, co-operative patient to perform a sustained activity and is therefore limited in its application. Tests commonly used include:

- lifting the head off the pillow for 5 seconds;
- a hand grip for 5 seconds;
- the ability to produce a vital capacity breath, >10 ml/kg.

In the patient who has not fully recovered from anaesthesia and has a reduced level of consciousness, residual neuromuscular block may be indicated by the presence of 'see-sawing' or paradoxical respiration.

In anaesthetized patients, a peripheral nerve stimulator is used, the details of which are outside the remit of this book. The following is intended as no more than a brief outline.

- A pair of cutaneous electrodes are used to stimulate a peripheral nerve which supplies a discrete muscle group and the resulting contractions observed or measured. One arrangement is to stimulate the ulnar nerve at the wrist whilst monitoring the contractions (twitch) of the adductor pollicis.
- Two sequences of stimulation are used:

  (i) approximately 50 mA, 0.2 seconds duration, repeated at 2 Hz for 2 seconds, giving a total of four stimuli, usually referred to as a 'train-of-four' (TOF);

  (ii) approximately 50 mA, 5 seconds duration, at 50 Hz, i.e. a tetanic stimulus.

- Following non-depolarizing neuromuscular blockade, there is a *progressive* decremental response to both types of stimuli, termed 'fade'. The ratio of the amplitude of the fourth twitch (T4) to the first twitch (T1) is used as an index of the degree of neuromuscular blockade. In addition, a tetanic stimulus preceding a TOF will result in 'facilitation' of the contractions compared with a pretetanic response, referred to as 'post-tetanic facilitation'.
- Following depolarizing blockade, the response to both types of stimulation is reduced but consistent, i.e. there is no fade or post-tetanic facilitation.

The peripheral nerve stimulator can be used:

- to distinguish between residual depolarizing and non-depolarizing block;
- to differentiate between apnoea due to prolonged action of suxamethonium, suggesting pseudocholinesterase deficiency or another cause, for example opioid overdose. The former will show reduced or absent response to stimulation, the latter a normal response;
- during long surgical procedures the timing of increments or the rate of

an infusion of relaxants can be adjusted to maintain a steady state and prevent sudden movement. This is particularly important during surgery in which a microscope is used, for example neurosurgery.

ANTICHOLINESTERASES

These are used to reverse non-depolarizing neuromuscular block by inhibiting the action of acetylcholinesterase, resulting in an increase in the concentration of acetylcholine. The speed of reversal of neuromuscular block will depend upon the intensity of block when reversal is attempted — the more intense the block the slower the reversal. They cannot be used to reverse very intense block, for example if given soon after the administration of a relaxant (no response to a TOF sequence).

Anticholinesterases also function at parasympathetic nerve endings (muscarinic effects), causing bradycardia, spasm of the bowel, bladder and bronchi, increased bronchial secretions, etc. Therefore they are always administered with a suitable dose of atropine or glycopyrrolate to block the unwanted muscarinic effects.

Neostigmine

A fixed dose of 2.5 mg intravenously is used in adults. Its maximal effect is seen after approximately 5 minutes and lasts for 20–30 minutes. It is usually administered concurrently with either atropine 1.2 mg or glycopyrrolate 0.5 mg.

Edrophonium

This is much less potent than neostigmine, with 0.5–1 mg/kg being required to ensure adequate reversal. Its muscarinic effects are claimed to be less severe than with neostigmine, its onset is faster and it is recommended that the patient should receive atropine a short time before the edrophonium.

MALIGNANT HYPERPYREXIA

In some individuals, exposure to certain anaesthetic drugs (typically suxamethonium and halothane) results in the release of abnormally high concentrations of calcium from the sarcoplasmic reticulum. This in turn causes increased muscle activity and metabolism and a progressive rise in body temperature due to an imbalance between heat production and loss.

Presentation

- An unexplained tachycardia.
- Tachypnoea in spontaneously breathing patients.
- Muscle rigidity, despite the use of relaxants.

- Failure to relax after suxamethonium.
- Cardiac dysrhythmias.
- A falling oxygen saturation and cyanosis.
- An increased end-tidal carbon dioxide.
- Labile blood pressure.

NB. It may go unnoticed unless the patient's temperature is being monitored.

Analysis of an arterial blood sample will demonstrate a profound metabolic acidosis (low pH and bicarbonate), a low Pao_2 and a high $Paco_2$. Continued muscle contraction results in hyperkalaemia and myoglobinaemia causing renal failure. Disseminated intravascular coagulation may develop, leading to consumption of coagulation factors and widespread haemorrhage.

Immediate management

1 The patient's airway is secured, and hyperventilation is started with 100% oxygen to compensate for the increased oxygen demand by muscle activity. All anaesthetic agents are stopped.

2 Active cooling is started with ice-cold 0.9% saline intravenously, and surface cooling by placing ice over axillary and femoral arteries.

3 Administer dantrolene intravenously. This is a calcium antagonist, specifically for use in the treatment of this condition.

4 Monitor temperature, heart rate, blood pressure, electrocardiogram (ECG), oxygen saturation Spo_2, end-tidal carbon dioxide, central venous pressure (CVP) and urine output.

Transfer the patient to the intensive care unit as soon as possible for continued monitoring, as their temperature may be labile for up to 48 hours.

Investigation of the family

Following an episode, the remainder of the patient's family are usually investigated for their susceptibility to malignant hyperpyrexia. This entails a muscle biopsy which is subjected to standardized contracture tests on exposure to halothane and caffeine. It is performed at specialized centres.

Anaesthesia for malignant hyperpyrexia susceptible patients

A regional anaesthetic technique using plain bupivacaine can be used, or alternatively a general anaesthesia avoiding triggering agents. A vapour-free machine and new circuits and hoses must be used. Those who have survived a previous episode or are known to be at risk may be pretreated with dantrolene (orally or intravenously).

Analgesics in anaesthesia

The sensory and emotional responses to the pain of surgery were originally eliminated by rendering patients unconscious using inhalational agents (e.g. ether, chloroform). Specific analgesic drugs are now used as part of the anaesthetic technique in all but the most minor of surgical procedures to eliminate the pain of surgery, reduce the autonomic response and allow the administration of lower concentrations of inhalational agents.

OPIOID ANALGESICS

This term is used to describe all drugs which have an analgesic effect mediated through opioid receptors and includes both naturally occurring and synthetic compounds. The term 'opiate' is now reserved for naturally occurring substances, for example morphine. Opioid drugs have either *agonist* or *antagonist* actions at opioid receptors. There are several receptors, each identified by a letter of the Greek alphabet, two of the most important being μ (mu) and κ (kappa). Stimulation of these receptors by a pure agonist produces the classical effects of opioids: analgesia (μ, κ), euphoria (μ), sedation (κ), depression of ventilation (μ, κ) and physical dependence (μ). The effects due to central and peripheral actions are summarized in Table 4.2.

Not all opioid analgesics are pure agonists. Some are partial agonists while others are mixed partial agonist/antagonist. At the other end of the spectrum are drugs which are pure antagonist and have no analgesic action. Such drugs will therefore reverse all the central actions of a pure agonist, and are used clinically in this role.

Because of the potential for physical dependence, there are strict rules governing the issue and use of most opioid drugs under the Misuse of Drugs Act 1971 (see below).

The pure opioid agonists

Morphine

Morphine is a natural extract of the opium poppy. It can be administered orally, intramuscularly, intravenously, subcutaneously, rectally, epidurally and intrathecally. It is most commonly used either intravenously 0.1–0.15 mg/kg (titrated in 1–2 mg increments) or intramuscularly 0.2–0.3 mg/kg. Analgesia occurs approximately 10–15 minutes after i.v. dose, 30–45 minutes after i.m. dose, and lasts 1–4 hours, the relatively slow onset being partly due to its low lipid solubility.

Morphine is effective against visceral pain, the pain of acute trauma

ACTIONS OF OPIOID DRUGS

Central nervous system
Analgesia
Sedation
Euphoria
Nausea and vomiting
Pupillary constriction
Depression of ventilation:
- rate more than depth
- reduced response to carbon dioxide

Depression of vasomotor centre
Addiction (not with normal clinical use)

Respiratory system
Antitussive effect
Bronchospasm in susceptible patients

Cardiovascular system
Peripheral venodilatation
Bradycardia due to vagal stimulation

Gastrointestinal tract
Reduced peristalsis causing:
- constipation
- delayed gastric emptying

Constriction of sphincters

Urinary tract
Increased sphincter tone and urinary retention

Skin
Itching

Endocrine system
Release of ADH and catecholamines

ADH, antidiuretic hormone.

Table 4.2 The actions of opioid drugs.

and the pain and anxiety of myocardial infarction. It is useful in left ventricular failure by causing venodilatation and reducing the sensation of dyspnoea.

Morphine is metabolized mainly by conjugation with glucuronic acid and is excreted via the kidneys.

The most important adverse actions of morphine are:

- nausea and vomiting as a result of stimulation of the chemoreceptor trigger zone on the floor of the fourth ventricle;
- respiratory depression due to a direct effect on the respiratory centre in the medulla;
- delayed gastric emptying and constipation due to reduced peristalsis;
- hypotension as a result of depression of the vasomotor centre and peripheral vasodilatation secondary to histamine release;
- increased sphincter tone leading to biliary spasm and retention of urine;
- cough suppression.

Diamorphine (heroin)

This is the *di*-acetyl ester of morphine. It is more lipid soluble, allowing rapid penetration of the blood–brain barrier where it is metabolized into monoacetyl morphine and morphine, which are the active components. Its main advantages over morphine are its greater potency and a more rapid rate of onset.

It is used in the management of chronic pain and is popular epidurally for acute pain relief. It is widely used in the management of acute myocardial infarction.

Fentanyl (Sublimaze)

This is a synthetic analgesic, and is widely used intraoperatively. It is a very lipid soluble, and is 80–100 times as potent as morphine.

It is most often used intravenously, but is occasionally administered intramuscularly as a premedicant. It is similar in its actions to morphine, apart from a more rapid onset of action, a greater degree of cardiovascular stability and more severe respiratory depression.

It is used over a wide range of dosages depending upon the clinical requirements:

- 1–3 µg/kg in spontaneously breathing patients or for short procedures, the duration of action being 30–40 minutes;
- 5–10 µg/kg in major procedures with controlled ventilation, for example cholecystectomy, total hip replacement;
- 50–100 µg/kg, producing sedation, unconsciousness and prolonged respiratory depression. Popular in cardiothoracic surgery because of the cardiovascular stability and frequent use of a period of elective ventilatory support immediately postoperatively.

Alfentanil (Rapifen)

This is related to fentanyl and has similar actions, but is only one fifth as potent. It has a very rapid onset, but a short duration of action as it is rapidly metabolized. It tends to be used either as an i.v. bolus dose of approximately 10 µg/kg for short procedures, or for longer procedures by continuous i.v. infusion of 0.5–2 µg/kg per minute with controlled ventilation. Even at small doses, it may cause marked respiratory depression in some patients. Its short duration of action makes it popular in day-case patients.

Sufentanil
One of the most potent synthetic analgesics, 6–7 times greater potency than fentanyl (600–700 times greater than morphine). Similar in its actions to fentanyl, but of shorter duration.

Remifentanil (Ultiva)
An ultra-short acting synthetic opioid analgesic as a result of its rapid metabolism by non-specific esterases. It has to be administered as a constant infusion and is increasingly popular as part of a TIVA technique (see page 64).

Pethidine
Pethidine has approximately one tenth the potency of morphine. It is used mainly for relief of pain postoperatively by i.m. injection at a dose of 1–2 mg/kg. It is shorter acting than morphine and associated with more nausea, vomiting and hypotension. There is less histamine release and it has less effect on the smooth muscle of sphincters which makes it popular after surgery on the gastrointestinal tract. It is metabolized in the liver to a variety of compounds which are excreted via the kidneys. Pethidine must not be given to patients taking monoamine oxidase inhibitors (see Table 1.6).

Papaveretum (Omnopon)
This is a mixture of alkaloids consisting predominantly of morphine with very small amounts of papaverine and codeine. It is available in two strengths containing the equivalent of 5 mg or 10 mg morphine and can be administered either intramuscularly or intravenously, but would seem to have little advantage over morphine alone.

The partial agonists and mixed agonist/antagonists
These drugs were introduced in the hope that, with only partial agonist activity at µ receptors or mixed agonist/antagonist actions at µ and κ receptors, analgesia would be achieved without the problem of depression of ventilation. Such an ideal has not yet been achieved.

Buprenorphine (Temgesic)

This is a synthetic compound related to morphine, but 30 times more potent. It is a partial agonist at μ receptors, which limits the analgesic effect even if the dose is increased (also called a 'ceiling' effect). It can be administered intravenously or intramuscularly at a dose of 0.3–0.6 mg or sublingually at a dose of 0.2 mg. It lasts up to 6–8 hours, and it may reduce the efficacy of any subsequently administered pure agonists such as morphine. It is similar to morphine in terms of side-effects, but ventilatory depression may be prolonged and difficult to reverse with naloxone (see below) due to its high receptor affinity. An alternative is to use doxapram, a specific respiratory stimulant. It has recently been added to the list of scheduled drugs because of increasing abuse.

Nalbuphine (Nubaine)

This is a synthetic analgesic with antagonist actions at μ receptors and partial agonist actions at κ receptors. It is similar in potency and duration of action to morphine, and exhibits a ceiling effect of analgesia (and depression of ventilation) like buprenorphine.

Tramadol (Zydol)

This is the most recently introduced synthetic analgesic and departs from the tradition of acting via one mechanism. Tramadol is both a weak opioid agonist at μ receptors and inhibits noradrenaline uptake and release of 5-hydroxytryptamine (5-HT). When given intravenously, it is approximately one tenth as potent as morphine and roughly equivalent to pethidine, i.e. the dose being 1–2 mg/kg. It is claimed to cause less respiratory depression than equivalent doses of morphine but if this does occur it is readily reversed by naloxone. A further advantage is that it is not a controlled drug, therefore making it more easily available.

The pure antagonist

The only one in common clinical use is naloxone.

Naloxone (Narcan)

This has antagonist actions at all the opioid receptors, reversing all the centrally mediated effects of pure opioid agonists. The initial i.v. dose in adults is 0.1–0.4 mg, which is effective in under 60 seconds and lasts for 30–45 minutes. It has a limited effect against those opioids with partial or mixed actions and complete reversal may require very high (10 mg) doses.

Following a severe overdose, either accidental or deliberate, several doses or an infusion of naloxone may be required as its duration of action is less than most opioids.

Interestingly, naloxone will also reverse the analgesia produced by acupuncture suggesting that this is probably mediated in part by the release of endogenous opioids.

THE REGULATION OF OPIOID DRUGS

As a result of the potential of opioid drugs for abuse and consequent physical dependence, their use in medicine is carefully regulated. The Misuse of Drugs Act 1971 controls 'dangerous or otherwise harmful drugs' which are designated 'Controlled Drugs' and includes the opioids. The act imposes a total prohibition on the manufacture, possession and supply of these substances in an attempt to prevent their misuse. The use of Controlled Drugs in medicine is permitted by the 'Misuse of Drugs Regulations 1985'. The drugs covered by these regulations are classified into five schedules, each with a different level of control.

• *Schedule 1:* hallucinogenic drugs including cannabis and LSD which currently have no recognized therapeutic use.

• *Schedule 2:* this includes opioids, major stimulants (amphetamines and cocaine) and quinalbarbitone.

• *Schedule 3:* drugs thought not as likely to be misused as those in schedule 2 and includes barbiturates, minor stimulants, buprenorphine (Temgesic) and temazepam.

• *Schedule 4:* benzodiazepines which are recognized as having the potential for abuse.

• *Schedule 5:* preparations which contain very low concentrations of codeine or morphine, for example cough mixtures.

Supply and custody of schedule 2 drugs

In the theatre complex, these drugs are supplied by the pharmacy, usually at the request of a senior member of the nursing staff in writing, specifying the drug, and the total quantity required and signed. These drugs must be stored in a locked safe, cabinet or room, constructed and maintained to prevent unauthorized access. A record must be kept of their use in the 'Controlled Drugs Register' and must comply with the following points:

• Separate parts of the register can be used for different drugs or strengths of drugs within a single class.

• The class of drug must be recorded at the head of each page.

• Entries must be in chronological sequence.

• Entries must be made on the day of the transaction or the next day.

• Entries must be in ink or otherwise indelible.

• No cancellation, alteration or obliteration may be made. Corrections must be accompanied by a footnote which must be dated.

- The register must not be used for any other purpose.
- A separate register may be used for each department (i.e. theatre).
- Registers must be kept for 2 years after the last dated entry.

The specific details required with respect to supply of Controlled Drugs (i.e. for the patient) are: the date of the transaction, name of person supplied (i.e. the patient's name), licence of person to be in possession (doctor's signature), amount supplied and form in which supplied.

NON-STEROIDAL ANTI-INFLAMMATORY DRUGS AS ANALGESICS

This group of drugs, usually referred to as NSAIDs, block the synthesis of prostaglandins by inhibition of the enzyme cyclo-oxygenase (prostaglandin synthetase). NSAIDs reduce pain by a peripheral action and centrally by reducing input of nociceptive information in the spinal cord. The degree of anti-inflammatory action compared with analgesic activity varies for the many different drugs available. Inhibition of prostaglandin synthesis is also responsible for the important side-effects of NSAIDs including: reduced platelet aggregation which may increase bleeding; damage to the gastric mucosa causing ulceration and bleeding; bronchospasm, particularly in allergic or atopic individuals; and reduced renal blood flow leading to renal failure. These actions tend to limit the usefulness of this group of drugs in anaesthesia and related areas.

Ketorolac

This is a NSAID with predominantly analgesic activity. The initial parenteral dose is 10 mg and subsequent doses of 30 mg (maximum 90 mg) for a maximum of 2 days. It is claimed to be as effective as morphine for pain relief after orthopaedic surgery and has opioid-sparing effects after abdominal surgery. As its actions are non-opioid, ketorolac has no effect on ventilation or cardiovascular function. It is not subject to the Misuse of Drugs Regulations.

As well as the usual contraindications to the use of NSAIDs, ketorolac should be avoided when excessive blood loss is anticipated, or when patients are receiving other NSAIDs or anticoagulants, including low-dose heparin.

Further reading

British Medical Association and the Royal Pharmaceutical Society of Great Britain. *British National Formulary*, September 1996, No. 32. London: British Medical Association and the Royal Pharmaceutical Society of Great Britain.

Brownlie GS, Walters FJM. Should we still be using nitrous oxide? *Current Anaesthesia and Critical Care* 1994; **5** (2): 109–14.

Buzello W. Muscle relaxants. *Current Opinion in Anesthesiology* 1993; **6** (4): 707–8.

Calvey TN, Williams NE. *Principles and Practice of Pharmacology for Anaesthetists*, 2nd edn. Oxford: Blackwell Scientific Publications, 1991.

Cashman JN. Volatile agents. In: Atkinson RS, Adams AP, eds. *Recent Advances in Anaesthesia and Analgesia*, No. 18. Edinburgh: Churchill Livingstone, 1994: 21–38.

Ingham JM, Portenoy RK. Drugs in the treatment of pain: NSAID's and opioids. *Current Opinion in Anesthesiology* 1993; **6** (5): 838–44.

Jones RM, Eger IE (eds). *Anaesthesia* 1995; **50**: 1–51 (Suppl.)

Meistelman C, McLoughlin C. Suxamethonium—current controversies. *Current Anaesthesia and Critical Care* 1993; **4** (1): 53–8.

Sebel PS. Opioids and other analgesics. *Current Opinion in Anesthesiology* 1993; **6** (4): 665–7.

CHAPTER 5

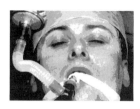

Measurement and Monitoring

Measurement and monitoring are closely linked but are not synonymous. A measuring instrument becomes a monitor when it is capable of delivering a warning when the variable being measured falls outside preset limits. The advent of modern electronics has turned many measuring devices into monitors. As a result of the contribution that monitoring has made to the reduction in morbidity and mortality in anaesthesia, guidelines have been introduced outlining the minimum safe requirements for patients undergoing anaesthesia. Not all patients require the same type or intensity of monitoring. What is used will depend upon a variety of factors including:

- the present and previous health of the patient;
- the type of operation and operative technique;
- the anaesthetic technique used;
- the equipment available and the anaesthetist's ability to use it;
- the preferences of the anaesthetist;
- any research being undertaken.

Monitoring is not without its own potential hazards. Faulty equipment may endanger the patient, for example from: (i) electrocution secondary to faulty earthing; (ii) the anaesthetist acting upon faulty data and instituting inappropriate treatment; and (iii) incorrect techniques to establish invasive monitoring. Ultimately, too many monitors may distract the anaesthetist from recognizing problems occurring in other areas.

Monitoring the cardiovascular system

Ideally one would wish to monitor the ability of the heart to maintain adequate perfusion of vital organs with oxygenated blood, but this is technically difficult and usually reserved for use during complex surgery or in very sick patients. Far more often, the adequacy of perfusion is assessed indirectly by monitoring the systemic blood pressure, the peripheral pulse, skin colour, temperature and urine output.

MEASUREMENT OF BLOOD PRESSURE

The blood pressure is a function of cardiac output *and* resistance to flow. It can be expressed as:

blood pressure = cardiac output × systemic vascular resistance.

Consequently, following haemorrhage, a patient may initially have a normal blood pressure, the fall in cardiac output being compensated for by an increase in the systemic vascular resistance (vasoconstriction), hence the patient has cold white hands and feet. In a septicaemic patient, the blood pressure may be low despite a high cardiac output, because of the pronounced vasodilatation seen as warm, pink extremities.

Blood pressure can be measured indirectly or directly.

Indirect

This is used during the vast majority of anaesthetics and is based upon the principle of gradual deflation of a pneumatic cuff placed around a limb, usually the upper arm. A cuff with a width that is *40% of the arm circumference* must be used and the internal inflatable bladder should encircle at least half the arm. If the cuff is too small for the arm, the blood pressure will be over-estimated, and if it is too large it will be under-estimated. Auscultation of the Korotkoff sounds is difficult in the operating theatre and automated methods, for example the Dinamap (Fig. 5.1), are now widely used. An electrical pump inflates the cuff which then undergoes controlled deflation. A microprocessor-controlled pressure transducer detects arterial wall motion and calculates systolic, mean and diastolic pressures,

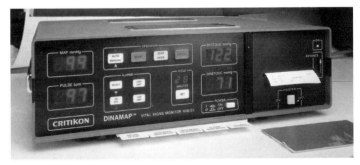

Fig. 5.1 Dinamap—non-invasive, automated blood pressure monitor. Courtesy of Johnson and Johnson Medical, Ascot, UK.

and heart rate. The frequency at which blood pressure is estimated can be set along with values for blood pressure outside which an alarm sounds. Such devices cannot measure pressure continuously and are less accurate at extremes of pressure and in patients with a dysrhythmia.

Direct

This is the most accurate method available for measuring blood pressure and is generally reserved for use in complex or prolonged surgery or sick patients. A cannula is inserted into a peripheral artery and connected to a transducer which turns the pressure signal to an electrical signal. This is then amplified and displayed as both a waveform and blood pressure (see Chapter 9).

PULSE AND PERIPHERAL PERFUSION

The pulse can be measured by direct palpation of a peripheral artery or by detecting the pulsatile flow through peripheral tissues (see Pulse oximetry). More often, the heart rate is derived from the electrocardiogram (ECG) signal (see below). As cardiac output falls, increasing vasoconstriction reduces the volume of the pulse and at extremes of vasoconstriction peripheral pulses may disappear altogether. At the same time, failing peripheral perfusion will be seen with gradual loss of skin colour and a decrease in peripheral skin temperature. A more accurate method of monitoring is to compare the core (nasopharyngeal or tympanic membrane) and peripheral (great toe) temperatures. Vasoconstriction maintains the core temperature at the expense of the periphery, therefore widening the gap.

THE ELECTROCARDIOGRAM

This is one of the most easily applied monitors and gives information on heart rate and rhythm, and may warn of the presence of ischaemia and acute disturbances of serum potassium and calcium concentrations. It is monitored using three of the standard limb leads (right arm, left arm and left leg) to give a tracing equivalent to standard lead II of the 12-lead ECG. For convenience, the electrodes are applied to the right shoulder (red), the left shoulder (yellow) and the left lower chest (green). An alternative is to place the electrodes on the manubrium, left shoulder and over the apex. This is called CM5 and is claimed to demonstrate the S-T segment more clearly, therefore being a better indicator of myocardial ischaemia. Some modern ECG monitors use five electrodes placed on the anterior chest so that all the standard leads can be displayed. Monitoring the ECG is now regarded as mandatory for all patients undergoing anaesthesia, irrespective of the length of the procedure. However, the ECG alone gives no information on the adequacy of the cardiac output and *it must be remembered that it is possible to have a virtually normal ECG in the absence of any cardiac output.*

URINE OUTPUT

Measurement of urine output is performed during prolonged surgery to ensure maintenance of adequate circulating volume where there is likely to be major blood loss, where diuretics are used (e.g. neurosurgery) and in all critically ill patients (catheterization also eliminates bladder overdistention or incontinence). Urine output needs to be measured at least hourly, aiming for a flow of approximately 1 ml/kg per hour. Failure to produce urine indicates that the renal blood flow is inadequate, as well as the flow to the other vital organs (heart and brain).

CENTRAL VENOUS PRESSURE

Starling's law of the heart states that 'the more the myocardial muscle fibres are stretched during diastole, the more forcibly they contract during systole and the more blood will be expelled'. The ventricular muscle fibres are stretched during diastole by the venous filling of the heart, which is termed the preload. Therefore, as preload increases, the output of each ventricle also increases. However, this phenomenon has an upper limit, beyond which further increases in muscle stretch (or preload) result in a smaller contraction (Fig. 5.2). Unfortunately, filling of the ventricles or preload cannot be measured easily, but a clinical estimate can be made by measuring the pressure in the ventricle at the end of diastole.

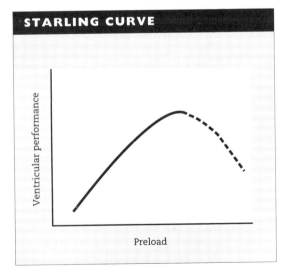

STARLING CURVE

Ventricular performance (y-axis)

Preload (x-axis)

Fig. 5.2 Graphical representation of Starling's law of the heart. The dashed line demonstrates the effect of overstretching.

When this is done for the right side of the heart it is termed the central venous pressure (CVP). Therefore, the CVP can be used as an index of the adequacy of diastolic filling and output of the right ventricle. Providing that there is no serious heart or lung disease (which may erroneously elevate the CVP), this can also be used to infer the adequacy of the output of the left ventricle.

Loss of circulating volume will reduce venous return to the heart, diastolic filling and preload, and will be reflected as a low or falling CVP. Although absolute values of the CVP can be measured, trends are usually more informative. Often a 'fluid challenge' is used in the face of a low CVP. The CVP is measured, a rapid infusion of fluid is given (3–5 ml/kg), and the change in CVP noted. In the hypovolaemic patient the CVP rises briefly and then rapidly falls to the previous value, whereas in the fluid replete patient the CVP will rise to a greater extent and be sustained.

CVP is usually measured in operations during which there is the potential for major fluid shifts (e.g. prolonged abdominal surgery) or blood loss (e.g. major orthopaedic and trauma surgery).

The CVP is also affected by a variety of other factors apart from fluid balance (Table 5.1), in particular the cardiac function. Failure of either ventricle will result in a back pressure and an elevation of the CVP. Hypotension in the presence of an elevated CVP (absolute or in response to a fluid challenge) may indicate heart failure, but most clinicians would now accept that measurement of the pressures on the left side of the heart using a pulmonary artery flotation catheter is preferable to assist in the management of this condition (see page 155).

FACTORS AFFECTING THE CVP

The zero reference point
Patient posture
Fluid status
Heart failure
Raised intrathoracic pressure:
- mechanical ventilation
- coughing
- straining

Pulmonary embolism
Pulmonary hypertension
Tricuspid valve disease
Pericardial effusion, tamponade
Superior vena cava obstruction

Table 5.1 Factors affecting the central venous pressure.

MEASURING BLOOD LOSS

Simple estimates of blood loss during surgery are easily performed. Swabs can be weighed, dry and wet, the increase in weight giving an indication of the amount of blood they have absorbed. The volume of blood in the suction apparatus can be measured, with allowance for irrigation fluids. Such methods are only estimates, as blood may remain in body cavities, be spilt on the floor and absorbed by drapes and gowns. In paediatric practice where small volumes of blood loss are relatively more important, all absorbent materials are washed to remove the blood and the resultant solvent assayed colorimetrically to estimate blood loss.

Monitoring the respiratory system

The main aims of monitoring the respiratory system are to ensure oxygenation and the elimination of carbon dioxide. Although these are now measured directly this should be supplemented by observation of the patient's colour, observing chest movement for rate, depth and symmetry, auscultation of the chest with a stethoscope and watching the reservoir bag on the anaesthetic system for rate and depth of breathing. During mechanical ventilation, airway pressure can be measured to avoid the risk of pulmonary barotrauma, to indicate obstruction to ventilation (e.g. bronchospasm, inadequate anaesthesia), or to indicate disconnection, with loss of pressure. The use of spirometry allows a comparison of inspiratory volume from the ventilator and expiratory volume from the patient and enables the identification of leaks.

OXYGENATION

All anaesthetic machines are fitted with a device warning of oxygen supply failure (see page 24). In addition, monitoring the inspired oxygen concentration is now regarded as essential for every anaesthetic (Fig. 5.3). The analyser should be positioned in the inspiratory limb, having been calibrated by prior exposure to air and 100% oxygen.

It must be remembered that the inspired oxygen concentration does not guarantee adequate arterial oxygen saturation as it may be insufficient to compensate for the effects of hypoventilation and ventilation/perfusion mismatch (see page 108).

PULSE OXIMETRY

The pulse oximeter consists of a probe, containing a light emitting diode (LED) and a photodetector, which can be applied across the tip of a digit or earlobe such that the light is transmitted through the tissues. The LED alternately transmits red light at two different wavelengths (in the visible

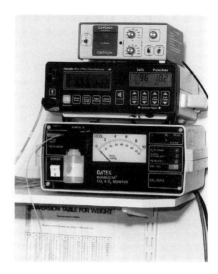

Fig. 5.3 (Top to bottom) Oxygen
analyser, pulse oximeter and
capnograph.

and infrared regions of the electromagnetic spectrum) which are
absorbed to different degrees by oxyhaemoglobin and deoxyhaemoglobin.
The intensity of transmitted light reaching the photodetector is converted
to an electrical signal. This information is processed and the absorption
due to the tissues and venous blood, which is static, is subtracted from the
beat-to-beat variation to display the peripheral arterial oxygen saturation
(Sp_{O_2}) both as a waveform and digital reading (see Fig. 5.3). Pulse oxime-
ters are accurate to $\pm 2\%$. The waveform can also be interpreted to give a
reading of heart rate. Alarms are provided for levels of saturation and
heart rate. Strictly speaking, the pulse oximeter relies on (and therefore
gives information about) both the circulatory and respiratory systems.

Advantages of the pulse oximeter

- Non-invasive.
- Provides continuous monitoring of oxygenation at tissue level.
- Unaffected by skin pigmentation.
- Portable, and mains or battery powered.

Disadvantages of the pulse oximeter

- Small changes in saturation result from large changes in Pa_{O_2}, above
90% because of the shape of the haemoglobin dissociation curve.
- Unreliable when there is severe vasoconstriction due to the reduced
pulsatile component of the signal.
- Unreliable with certain haemoglobins:

(a) when carboxyhaemoglobin is present, it overestimates SaO_2;
(b) when methaemoglobin is present, at an $SaO_2 > 85\%$, it underestimates the saturation.

- Progressively under-reads the saturation as the haemoglobin falls (but it is not affected by polycythaemia).
- May be affected by extraneous light.
- May be unreliable when there is excessive movement of the patient.

> The pulse oximeter is not an indicator of the adequacy of alveolar ventilation. Hypoventilation can be compensated for by increasing the inspired oxygen concentration, to maintain oxygen saturation.

Despite these limitations, the pulse oximeter is now regarded by many as the single most useful monitor and they are used in several areas outside anaesthesia, for example during prehospital care and transport of critically ill patients.

THE ELIMINATION OF CARBON DIOXIDE

Carbon dioxide (CO_2) is measured using a capnograph (see Fig. 5.3), util-

---

END-TIDAL CARBON DIOXIDE

1 An indicator of the degree of alveolar ventilation:
   - to ensure normocapnia during mechanical ventilation
   - control the level of hypocapnia in neurosurgery
   - avoidance of hypocapnia where the cerebral circulation is impaired, e.g. the elderly
2 As a disconnection indicator if the reading suddenly falls to zero
3 To indicate that the tracheal tube is in the trachea
4 As an indicator of the degree of rebreathing (presence of carbon dioxide in inspired gas), e.g. using a Bain system
5 As an indicator of cardiac output. If cardiac output falls and ventilation is maintained, then end-tidal carbon dioxide falls as carbon dioxide is not delivered to the lungs, e.g.:
   - hypovolaemia
   - cardiac arrest, where it can also be used to indicate effectiveness of external cardiac compression
   - massive pulmonary embolus
6 It may be the first clue of the development of malignant hyperpyrexia (see page 69)

Table 5.2 Uses of end-tidal carbon dioxide measurement.

izing the property that carbon dioxide absorbs infrared light. In a healthy person, the carbon dioxide concentration in alveolar gas (or partial pressure, PA_{CO_2}) correlates well with partial pressure in arterial blood (Pa_{CO_2}), with the former being slightly lower by 5 mmHg or 0.7 kPa. Alveolar gas is best represented by analysing gas at end expiration and therefore *end-tidal carbon dioxide* concentration is measured. This is inversely proportional to alveolar ventilation and it is measured primarily as an indicator of the adequacy of ventilation. Modern capnographs have alarms for when the end-tidal carbon dioxide is outside preset limits. Other uses of carbon dioxide monitoring are given in Table 5.2.

> The gap between arterial and end-tidal carbon dioxide is increased (end-tidal falls) in sick patients, mainly due to the development of increased areas of ventilation/perfusion mismatch and in those with chest disease due to poor mixing of respiratory gases.

Miscellaneous

INHALATIONAL AGENTS

The inspired or end-tidal concentration of these agents can be measured using infrared absorption, similar to carbon dioxide. Absorption varies between agents and their concentration, and a single device can be calibrated for all of the commonly used agents.

TEMPERATURE

During anaesthesia patients cool as a result of exposure to a cold environment, evaporation of fluids from body cavities, breathing dry, cold anaesthetic gases, and the administration of cold intravenous fluids. This is compounded by the loss of body temperature regulation and inability to shiver. Appropriate preventative measures should be taken to minimize the above: placing the patient on a warming mattress, warming cold fluids (particularly blood), heating and humidifying inspired gases, and covering exposed areas. The effectiveness of these methods can be monitored by measuring the patient's temperature in the oesophagus (cardiac temperature) and nasopharynx (brain temperature) using a thermistor, the resistance of which is temperature dependent. Alternatively, an infrared tympanic membrane thermometer can be used which gives a good indication of brain temperature. The rectum can be used, but faeces may insulate the thermistor leading to inaccuracies. Apart from monitoring heat loss, a sudden unexpected rise in a patient's temperature may be the first warning of the development of malignant hyperpyrexia (see page 69).

DISCONNECT ALARMS

Whenever a patient is being mechanically ventilated, a disconnect alarm should be used. They are pressure sensitive and detect whenever the airway pressure has failed to reach a predetermined level after a fixed interval. They can also be used to detect high airway pressures, caused, for example, by obstruction or the patient coughing.

Monitoring neuromuscular blockade is covered in Chapter 4. Many other physiological parameters can be, and are, monitored during anaesthesia when appropriate. Some examples are: clotting profiles in patients receiving a transfusion of a large volume of stored blood, blood glucose in diabetic patients and arterial blood gas and acid–base analysis during the bypass phase of cardiac surgery. Recently, interest has been shown in the development of monitors which give information relating to the depth of anaesthesia, but these are still under investigation.

THE ANAESTHETIC RECORD

On every occasion an anaesthetic is administered, a comprehensive and *legible* record must be made. The details and method of recording will vary with each case, the type of chart used and the equipment available. Apart from the value to future anaesthetists who encounter the patient, particularly when there has been a difficulty (e.g. with intubation), the anaesthetic record is a medicolegal document, to which reference may be necessary after several years. An anaesthetic chart typically allows the following to be recorded:

- preoperative findings, ASA grade (American Society of Anesthesiologists), premedication;
- details of previous anaesthetics and any difficulties;
- apparatus used for the current anaesthetic;
- monitoring devices used;
- anaesthetic and other drugs administered: timing, dose and route;
- vital signs at various intervals, usually on a graphical section;
- fluids administered and lost: type and volume;
- use of local or regional anaesthetic techniques;
- anaesthetic difficulties or complications;
- postoperative instructions.

Further reading

The Association of Anaesthetists of Great Britain and Ireland *Recommendations for Stan-*

dards of Monitoring during Anaesthesia and Recovery. London: The Association of Anaesthetists of Great Britain and Ireland, 1988.

Ralston AC, Webb RK, Runciman WB. Potential errors in pulse oximetry: I. Pulse oximeter evaluation. *Anaesthesia* 1991; **46**: 202–6.

Webb RK, Ralston AC, Runciman WB. Potential errors in pulse oximetry: II. Effects of changes in saturation and signal quality. *Anaesthesia* 1991; **46**: 207–12.

Winter A, Spence AA. An international consensus on monitoring? *British Journal of Anaesthesia* 1990; **64**: 263–6.

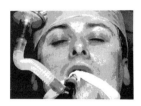

Intravenous Cannulation and Fluid Administration

Intravenous (i.v.) cannulation can be achieved in several ways. The most common technique is by percutaneous puncture of a peripheral vein using a cannula mounted on a metal needle. Central veins are frequently cannulated using the Seldinger technique, whereas during resuscitation an alternative is to surgically expose a vein and insert a cannula under direct vision —the 'cutdown' technique. Intravenous cannulation in anaesthesia is used:
- for the administration of drugs for the induction and maintenance of anaesthesia;
- for the administration of fluids to maintain or restore the patient's circulation;
- to monitor intravascular pressures.

Peripheral intravenous cannulation

The veins most commonly used during anaesthesia are the superficial peripheral veins in the upper limbs. Cannulation of the central veins is a technique usually used for monitoring patients.

ANATOMY OF THE VEINS USED FOR INTRAVENOUS ACCESS

The dorsum of the hand and forearm

These are the veins most commonly used by anaesthetists. The veins draining the fingers unite to form three *dorsal metacarpal veins*. Laterally these are joined by veins from the thumb and continue up the radial border of the forearm as the *cephalic vein* (Fig. 6.1). Medially the metacarpal veins unite with the veins from the little finger and pass up the ulnar border of the forearm as the *basilic vein*. There is often a large vein in

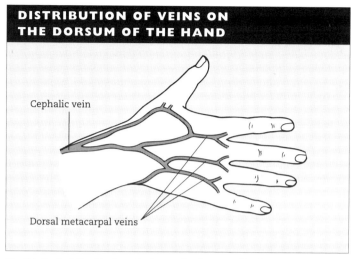

DISTRIBUTION OF VEINS ON THE DORSUM OF THE HAND

Cephalic vein

Dorsal metacarpal veins

Fig. 6.1 Typical distribution of veins on the dorsum of the hand. After Warwick R & Williams PL (eds) *Gray's Anatomy*, 35th edn. Edinburgh: Churchill Livingstone, 1973.

the middle of the ventral (anterior) aspect of the forearm — the *median vein of the forearm* (Fig. 6.2).

The antecubital fossa

The cephalic vein passes through the antecubital fossa on the lateral side and the basilic vein enters the antecubital fossa very medially, just in front of the medial epicondyle of the elbow. These veins are joined by the *median cubital* or *antecubital vein*. The median vein of the forearm also drains into the basilic vein (see Fig. 6.2). Veins in this region tend to be used only when attempts to cannulate the above veins have failed. The proximity of other structures, for example the brachial artery, the median nerve and branches of the medial and lateral cutaneous nerves of the arm, are easily damaged by needles or extravasated drugs.

EQUIPMENT

A variety of devices of different lengths and diameters are used. The term 'cannula' is used for those of 7 cm or less in length and 'catheter' for those longer than 7 cm. The outside diameter of the device is often quoted in terms of its 'gauge'. The diameter increases with decreasing gauge. Increasingly, the external diameter is now quoted in millimetres. Three main types of cannulae can be used to secure venous cannulation.

I *Butterfly type.* A short metal needle with two flexible plastic wings

DISTRIBUTION OF VEINS OF THE FOREARM AND ANTECUBITAL FOSSA (RIGHT ARM)

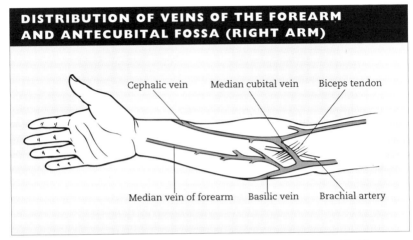

Fig. 6.2 Typical distribution of veins of the forearm and antecubital fossa (right arm). After Warwick R & Williams PL (eds) *Gray's Anatomy*, 35th edn. Edinburgh: Churchill Livingstone, 1973.

attached (Fig. 6.3A). As the cannula is entirely metal it can tear the vein if it moves about, resulting in loss of access, haemorrhage and potential damage to surrounding structures. Because of these risks it will not be considered further.

2 *Cannula over needle.* This is by far the most popular device and is available in a wide variety of sizes, 12–27 gauge. A plastic (PTFE or similar material) cannula is mounted on a smaller diameter metal needle, the bevel of which protrudes from the cannula. The other end of the needle is attached to a transparent 'flashback chamber', which fills with blood once the needle bevel lies within the vein (Fig. 6.3B). Some devices have flanges or 'wings' to facilitate attachment to the skin (Fig. 6.3C, D). All cannulae have a standard Luer-lock fitting for attaching a giving set and some have a valved injection port through which drugs can be administered (Fig. 6.3D).

3 *Seldinger type.* This is used predominantly to achieve cannulation of the central veins, but peripheral devices are now available, designed mainly for use in fluid resuscitation (e.g. Arrow EID cannula) (Fig. 6.3E).

Fluid flow through cannulae and catheters is determined by four factors.

1 *Internal diameter.* Flow is theoretically proportional to the fourth power of the radius. Doubling the diameter should result in flow increasing 16-fold (2^4). This is rarely achieved in practice, but an increase of four- to fivefold will be seen.

2 *Length.* Flow is inversely proportional to the length of the cannula — doubling the length will halve the flow.

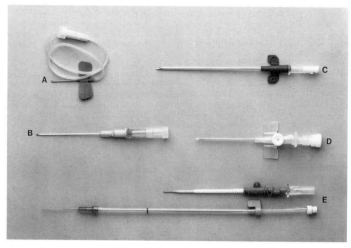

Fig. 6.3 (A–E) Various intravenous cannulae. Courtesy of Greaves I, Hodgetts T, Porter K. *Emergency Care—A Textbook for Paramedics*. London: Harcourt Brace, 1997.

3   *Viscosity.* Flow is inversely proportional to the viscosity of the fluid—increasing viscosity reduces flow. Colloids and blood flow much more slowly than a crystalloid, particularly when they are cold.
4   *Pressure.* Increasing the pressure across the cannula will increase the flow. This is usually achieved by either raising the height of the drip above the patient or using external pressure.

> During resuscitation the rate of flow is determined primarily by the diameter of the cannula, therefore always use short, wide-bore ones.

TECHNIQUE FOR CANNULATION OF A PERIPHERAL VEIN

The superficial veins are situated immediately under the skin in the superficial fascia, along with a variable amount of subcutaneous fat. The veins are relatively mobile and capable of considerable variation in their diameter. The size of cannula used will depend upon its purpose: large-diameter cannulas are required for rapid fluid administration, smaller ones are required if simply for drug administration.

> As with any procedure where there is a risk of contact with body fluids, gloves should be worn by the operator.

1   Choose a vein capable of accommodating the size of cannula needed, preferably one that is both visible and palpable. The junction of two veins is often a good site as the 'target' is relatively larger. Avoid veins over joints as the cannula may kink if the joint is flexed and function may be lost. Veins distal to fractures should also be avoided as drugs or fluids will leak from the fracture site. Encourage the vein to dilate by using a tourniquet and gently tapping the skin over the vein. Warming a cold hand will also help.

2   Clean the skin over the vein using either an alcohol- or iodine-based solution (ensure there is no risk of allergy if iodine is used). A small amount of local anaesthetic (0.2 ml lignocaine 1%) should be infiltrated into the skin at the site chosen for venepuncture using a 22–25 gauge needle, particularly if a large (>1.2 mm, 18 gauge) cannula is used. This reduces the pain of cannulation and makes the patient less likely to move and less resistant to further attempts. If a large cannula is used, insertion through the skin may be facilitated by first making a small incision with either a 19 gauge needle or a scalpel blade, taking care not to puncture the vein.

3   Immobilize the vein by pulling the skin over the vein tight, using the operator's spare hand (Fig. 6.4). This prevents it being displaced by the cannula. Advance the cannula through the skin at an angle of 10–15° and then into the vein. Often a slight loss of resistance is felt as the vein is entered and this should be accompanied by the appearance of blood in the flashback chamber of the cannula (Fig. 6.5). This indicates that only the tip of the needle is within the vein.

4   Reduce the angle of the cannula and advance it a further 2–3 mm into the vein, keeping the skin taut. This ensures that the first part of the plastic cannula lies within the vein. Care must be taken at this point not to push the needle out of the far side of the vein. Withdraw the needle 5–10 mm

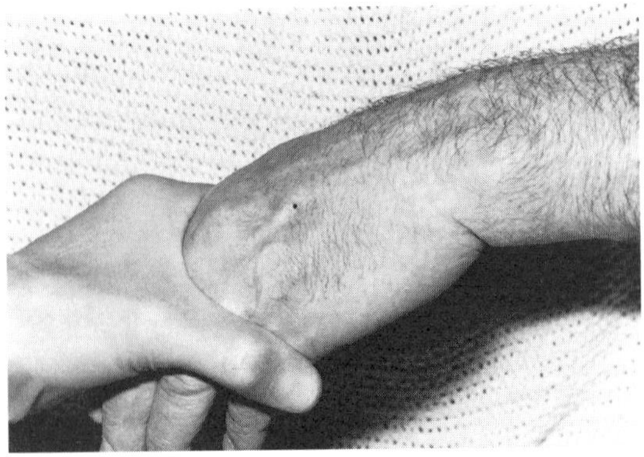

Fig. 6.4 Vein immobilized, dilated and ready for cannulation. Courtesy of Greaves I, Hodgetts T, Porter K. *Emergency Care—A Textbook for Paramedics.* London: Harcourt Brace, 1997.

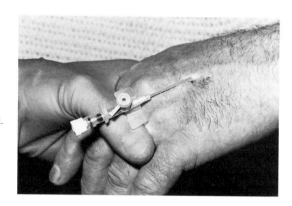

Fig. 6.5 Cannula inserted showing flashback of blood. Courtesy of Greaves I, Hodgetts T, Porter K. *Emergency Care—A Textbook for Paramedics*. London: Harcourt Brace, 1997.

into the cannula so that the bevel no longer protrudes from the end. Often as this is done, blood will be seen to flow between the needle body and the cannula, confirming that the tip of the cannula is within the vein (Fig. 6.6).

5   The cannula and needle should now be advanced together along the vein. The needle is retained within the cannula to provide support and prevent kinking at the point of skin puncture (Fig. 6.7). Once the cannula is fully inserted, the tourniquet should be released, and the needle completely removed and disposed of safely.

6   Confirmation that the cannula lies within the vein can be made by attaching an i.v. infusion and ensuring that it runs freely, or by injecting a small volume of saline. Immediate, localized swelling or pain indicates that the cannula is incorrectly positioned.

7   Finally, secure the cannula in an appropriate manner with adhesive tape, or a commercial dressing.

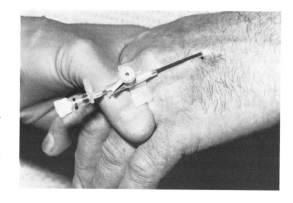

Fig. 6.6 Cannula with needle slightly withdrawn. Courtesy of Greaves I, Hodgetts T, Porter K. *Emergency Care—A Textbook for Paramedics*. London: Harcourt Brace, 1997.

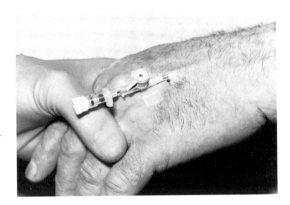

Fig. 6.7 Cannula fully inserted. Courtesy of Greaves I, Hodgetts T, Porter K. *Emergency Care—A Textbook for Paramedics.* London: Harcourt Brace, 1997.

COMPLICATIONS

Most are relatively minor but this must not be used as an excuse for carelessness and poor technique.

Early complications

- *Failed cannulation:* usually a result of pushing the needle completely through the vein. It is always best to cannulate a distal vein in a limb and work proximally. If further attempts are required, fluid or drugs will not leak from previous puncture sites.
- *Haematoma:* usually secondary to the above with inadequate pressure applied over the puncture site to prevent bleeding. They are made worse by forgetting to remove the tourniquet!
- *Extravasation of fluid or drugs:* often a result of failing to recognize that the cannula is not within the vein before use. Placing a cannula over a joint, or prolonged use to infuse fluids under pressure, also predispose to leakage. Damage to the overlying tissues will depend primarily upon the nature of the extravasated fluid.
- *Damage to local structures:* secondary to poor technique and lack of knowledge of the local anatomy.
- *Air embolus:* rare as the peripheral veins collapse when empty. However, a cannula may prevent this and allow air to enter the circulation. It is most likely to happen in the central veins, particularly if the patient is in a head-up position.
- *Shearing of the cannula:* usually as a result of trying to reintroduce the needle after it has been withdrawn. The safest action is to withdraw the whole cannula and attempt cannulation at another site.

Late complications

- *Thrombophlebitis:* related to the length of time the vein is in use and irritation caused by the substances flowing through it. High concentrations of drugs and fluids with extremes of pH or high osmolality are the main causes, for example calcium chloride, sodium bicarbonate and antibiotics. Once a vein shows signs of thrombophlebitis (i.e. tender, red and deteriorating flow) the cannula must be removed to prevent subsequent infection or thrombosis which may spread proximally.

Central venous cannulation

Cannulation of the central veins may be used for a wide variety of reasons during anaesthesia — to monitor the cardiovascular system, because of inadequate peripheral venous access and to administer certain drugs (e.g. inotropes). There are many different types of equipment and approaches to the central veins, and the following is intended simply as an outline.

EQUIPMENT FOR CENTRAL VENOUS CATHETERIZATION

Three types of catheter are commonly used for percutaneous cannulation of the central veins.

1 *Catheter over needle.* These are similar to a peripheral i.v. cannula and are inserted using the same technique. The main difference is that the catheter is longer to ensure that the tip lies in the correct position within a central vein.

2 *Seldinger technique.* The chosen vein is initially punctured percutaneously using a small-diameter needle. A flexible guidewire is then passed down the needle into the vein and the needle carefully withdrawn, leaving the wire behind. The catheter is now passed over the wire into the vein, sometimes preceded by a dilator. The advantage of this method is that the initial use of a small needle increases the chance of successful venepuncture and reduces the risk of damage to the vein.

3 *Catheter through needle.* A large-diameter needle is introduced into the vein, the catheter is threaded down the lumen and the needle is withdrawn leaving the catheter in place.

ACCESS TO THE CENTRAL VEINS

Peripheral veins can be used to access the central veins, but the larger veins around the neck are more popular routes. Occasionally the femoral vein may be used.

Veins in the antecubital fossa

The basilic vein is preferable, as a catheter passed along the cephalic vein frequently fails to reach beyond the clavipectoral fascia. This route of inserting a central venous pressure (CVP) catheter has only a 60% success rate, but this must be offset against this method's relatively few

COMPLICATIONS OF CVP CATHETER

Arterial puncture and bleeding causing haematoma or haemothorax
Air embolus
Venous thrombosis
Pneumothorax
Thoracic duct injury (left side) and chylothorax
Hydrothorax if the catheter is intrapleural and fluid given
Bacteraemia
Septicaemia
Injury to nerves:
    brachial plexus
    recurrent laryngeal
    phrenic
Soft tissue infection at puncture site

Table 6.1 Complications of inserting CVP catheter.

complications, the most important of which is thrombophlebitis after prolonged use (>48 hours).

The internal jugular vein

The right internal jugular offers certain advantages: there is a 'straight line'
to the heart, the apical pleura does not rise as high on this side, and the
main thoracic duct is on the left. The internal jugular approach is associated with the highest incidence of success (95%), and a low rate of complications (Table 6.1).

Subclavian vein

This can be approached by both the supra- and infraclavicular routes. Both
are technically more difficult than the internal jugular route and there is a
significant incidence of causing a pneumothorax ($\approx$5%). The main advantage of this route is comfort for the patient during long-term use.

Bilateral attempts at central venous cannulation must not be made
because of the risk of airway obstruction due to haematoma formation in
the neck or bilateral pneumothoraces.

> Whenever a CVP catheter is inserted, a chest X-ray should be taken
> to ensure that a pneumothorax has not been caused and that the
> catheter is correctly positioned.

Intravenous fluids

During anaesthesia, i.v. fluids are used to provide the patient's normal daily requirements and replace losses due to surgery. Three types of fluid are used: crystalloids, colloids, and blood and its components.

CRYSTALLOIDS

These are solutions of crystalline solids in water. A wide variety are available for use and a summary of the composition of the most commonly used is shown in Table 6.2. Those containing sodium in similar concentrations to plasma are rapidly distributed throughout the extracellular fluid space (i.e. intravascular and interstitial volumes). Ultimately, only 25–30% of the volume administered remains intravascular. If used to restore the circulating volume, approximately three times the deficit will need to be given. If crystalloids are used which contain a lower concentration of sodium than plasma (e.g. 4% glucose plus 0.18% saline), then once the glucose is metabolized, the remaining fluid is distributed throughout the entire body water (i.e. extracellular and intracellular volumes), and even less will remain intravascular, as little as 10%. These fluids are used primarily to provide a patient's daily requirements of water and sodium and are frequently referred to as 'maintenance fluids'.

COLLOIDS

These are suspensions of high molecular weight particles. A wide variety are available, the most commonly used are derived from gelatin (Haemaccel, Gelofusine), protein (albumin) or starch (Hespan). A summary of their

COMPOSITION OF CRYSTALLOIDS

Crystalloid	Na^+ (mmol/l)	K^+ (mmol/l)	Ca^{2+} (mmol/l)	Cl^- (mmol/l)	HCO_3^- (mmol/l)	pH	Osmolality (mosmol/l)
Hartmann's solution	131	5	4	112	29*	6.5	281
0.9% sodium chloride	154	0	0	154	0	5.5	300
4% glucose plus 0.18% sodium chloride	31	0	0	31	0	4.5	284
5% glucose	0	0	0	0	0	4.1	278

*Present as lactate which is metabolized to bicarbonate by the liver.

Table 6.2 Composition of commonly used crystalloids.

COMPOSITION OF COLLOIDS

Colloid	Na$^+$ (mmol/l)	K$^+$ (mmol/l)	Ca^{2+} (mmol/l)	Cl$^-$ (mmol/l)	HCO$_3^-$ (mmol/l)	pH	Osmolality (mosmol/l)
Haemaccel	145	5	6.2	145	0	7.3	350
Gelofusine	154	0.4	0.4	125	0	7.4	465
Albumin	130–160	2	0	120	0	6.7–7.3	270–300
Starch	154	0	0	154	0	5.5	310

Table 6.3 Composition of commonly used colloids.

composition is shown in Table 6.3. Colloids are not lost into the remainder of the extracellular or intracellular volume. They primarily expand the intravascular volume and can be administered in a volume similar to the deficit to maintain the circulating volume. They have a finite life in the plasma and will eventually be either metabolized or excreted.

BLOOD AND BLOOD COMPONENTS

There are several forms of blood and its components available. In the intraoperative period the most commonly used are red cell products, platelet concentrates and clotting factors.

Red cell products

- *Whole blood*. Despite its name, this is basically red cells, plasma proteins and clotting factors (levels of V and VIII are low). There are no platelets. Each unit contains approximately 510 ml with a haematocrit of 35–45%.
- *Red cell concentrate*. This is the by-product of the removal of plasma from whole blood. Each unit contains 250 ml with a haematocrit of 60–75% and is hence very viscous with a poor flow rate.
- *Red cells in optimal additive solution*. A red cell concentrate to which a mixture of saline, adenine and glucose has been added. This improves both red cell survival and flow characteristics. Each unit contains 300 ml with a haematocrit of 50–70%.

Platelet concentrates

These are supplied as either individually donated units or as a pack containing a pool of four to six donor units. Each pack contains 50–60 ml and 55×10^9 platelets. Four to six units are normally administered rapidly (<30 minutes) via a fresh standard giving set *without* the use of a microaggregate filter, as these result in the loss of significant numbers of platelets.

Clotting factors

- *Fresh frozen plasma (FFP)*. This consists of the plasma separated from a single donation and frozen within 6 hours. Each pack contains 200–250 ml, with normal levels of clotting factors (except factor VIII, 70% normal). It should be infused as soon as it has thawed.
- *Cryoprecipitate*. This is produced as a precipitate formed on the controlled thawing of FFP, which is collected and suspended in plasma. It contains large amounts of factor VIII and fibrinogen. It is supplied as a pooled donation from six packs of FFP in one unit and must be used as soon as possible after thawing.

Risks of intravenous blood and blood products

All blood donations are routinely tested for hepatitis B surface antigen, antibodies to the human immunodeficiency virus (HIV) and hepatitis C. However, a period exists between exposure and the development of antibodies. The resultant infected red cells would not be detected by current screening techniques. The risk is very small and has been estimated for hepatitis B at $1:10^5$ and for HIV at $1:10^6$ units transfused. In order to try and eliminate these risks, techniques now exist for using the patient's own blood in the perioperative period.

- *Predepositing blood*. Over a period of 4 weeks prior to surgery, the patient builds up a bank of two to four units of blood which can be retransfused during surgery.
- *Preoperative haemodilution*. Immediately prior to surgery, between 0.5 and 1.5 l of blood is removed and replaced with colloid. This is then retransfused at the end of surgery, providing the patient with fresh blood.
- *Cell savers*. These devices collect blood lost during surgery via a suction system, the red cells are separated, washed and resuspended ready for retransfusion to the patient.

Intraoperative fluid administration

The type and volume of fluid administered during surgery varies for each and every patient, but has to take into account the following: (i) any deficit the patient has accrued; (ii) maintenance requirements during the procedure; (iii) losses due to surgery; and (iv) any vasodilatation secondary to the use of a regional anaesthetic technique (see page 144).

THE ACCRUED DEFICIT

This may be due to preoperative fasting, or losses as a result of vomiting, haemorrhage or pyrexia. The deficits due to fasting are predominantly water from the total body water volume. The volume required is calculated at the normal daily maintenance rate of 1.5 ml/kg per hour (from the point at which fasting began). Although this deficit can be replaced with a fluid such as 4% glucose plus 0.18% saline, it is not uncommon to find Hartmann's solution used intraoperatively. The other main cause of a preoperative deficit is losses either from or into the gastrointestinal tract. This fluid usually contains electrolytes and effectively depletes the extracellular volume. It is best replaced with a crystalloid of similar composition, particularly in respect of the sodium concentration. Either 0.9% sodium chloride or Hartmann's solution is used.

Acute blood loss preoperatively can be replaced with either an appropriate volume of crystalloid (remembering that only 30% remains intravascular) or colloid. If more than 20% of the estimated blood volume has been lost (approximately 1000 ml), blood should be used, particularly if bleeding is ongoing.

INTRAOPERATIVE REQUIREMENTS

Maintenance fluids alone are usually only administered where surgery is prolonged (>2 hours), or where there is the possibility of a delay in the patient resuming oral fluid intake. Most patients will compensate for a preoperative deficit by increasing their oral intake postoperatively. When a maintenance fluid is used it should be administered at 1.5 ml/kg per hour, and increased if the patient is pyrexial by 10% for each degree centigrade above normal.

Losses due to surgery occur in three main ways.

1   *Evaporation:* during body cavity surgery or when large areas of tissue are exposed, depleting the total body water.

2   *Trauma:* resulting in the formation of tissue oedema, the volume of which is dependent upon the extent of tissue damage and similar in composition to extracellular fluid. This fluid is often referred to as 'third space loss' and creates a deficit in the circulating volume as the volume can no longer be accessed.

3   *Blood loss:* the volume of which will depend upon the type of surgery and the site where it is being performed.

Fluid losses from the first two causes are difficult to measure and are extremely variable. If evaporative losses are considered excessive then 4% glucose plus 0.18% saline can be used. Third space losses should be replaced with a solution similar in composition to extracellular fluid and Hartmann's is commonly used. The rate of administration and volume required is proportional to surgical trauma and may be as much as 10 ml/kg per hour. Blood pressure, pulse, peripheral perfusion and urine output will give an indication as to the adequacy of replacement, but in complex cases where there are other causes of fluid loss, particularly bleeding, the measurement of the CVP is very useful (see page 82).

Blood loss is slightly more obvious and easier to measure. Most previously well patients will tolerate the anaemia that results from the loss of 20% of their blood volume, providing that the circulating volume is adequately maintained by the use of crystalloids or colloids. Beyond this, red cell preparations are used in order to maintain the oxygen carrying capacity of the blood and usually achieved by aiming for a haematocrit of around 30% (a haemoglobin of 100 g/l).

In most cases, the equivalent of the patient's estimated blood volume can be replaced with red cell concentrates, crystalloid and colloid in the appropriate volumes. Occasionally, blood loss is such that the haemostatic mechanisms are affected. This may be seen as continuous oozing from the surgical wound, around i.v. cannulation sites and bleeding from mucous membranes. This can be dealt with by the use of either whole blood or a combination of red cell concentrate and FFP. Platelets may not be required until losses exceed 1.5 times the estimated blood volume. When circumstances such as these arise, therapy is best directed by the results of laboratory investigations rather than being administered blindly. Treatment is usually reserved for those cases in which the INR (prothrombin time ratio) reaches 1.7–2.0, fibrinogen levels fall below 0.5 g/l or the platelet count falls below $50 \times 10^9/l$.

Further reading

Driscoll PA, Gwinnutt CL, Mackway-Jones K, Wardle T (eds). *Advanced Cardiac Life Support—The Practical Approach*, 2nd edn. London: Chapman & Hall, in press.

Evans RJ, McCabe M, Thomas R. Intraosseous infusion. *British Journal of Hospital Medicine* 1994; 51: 161–4.

Rosen M, Latto IP, Ng WS. *Handbook of Percutaneous Central Venous Catheterisation*. London: WB Saunders Co, 1981.

Soni N (ed.). Intravascular access. *Practical Procedures in Anaesthesia and Intensive Care*. Oxford: Butterworth Heinemann, 1989.

Tonks A. How to put up a drip. *Student British Medical Journal* 1992; 1: 57.

United Kingdom Health Departments. *Handbook of Transfusion Medicine*. London: Her Majesty's Stationery Office, 1989.

Warwick R, Williams PL (eds). Chapter 6: Angiology. *Gray's Anatomy*, 35th edn. Edinburgh: Churchill Livingstone, 1973; 588–744.

CHAPTER 7

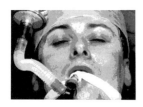

Postanaesthesia Care

For the vast majority of patients, recovery from anaesthesia and surgery is uneventful. However, an unpredictable proportion of patients will suffer early complications and it is now accepted that all patients recovering from anaesthesia should be nursed in an area with appropriate facilities to deal with any of the problems which may arise, and by trained staff.

The recovery area

All patients should be recovered on a tipping trolley unless a prolonged stay is expected, when they may be recovered on their bed. Each recovery bay should be equipped with:

- an oxygen supply plus appropriate circuits for administration;
- suction;
- an electrocardiogram (ECG) monitoring device;
- a pulse oximeter;
- a non-invasive blood pressure monitor.

In addition the following must be immediately available:

• *Airway equipment:* oral and nasal airways, a range of endotracheal tubes, laryngoscopes, a bronchoscope and the instruments to perform a cricothyroidotomy and tracheostomy.

• *Breathing and ventilation equipment:* self-inflating bag-valve-masks, a mechanical ventilator and a chest drain set.

• *Circulation:* a defibrillator, drugs for cardiopulmonary resuscitation, a range of intravenous (i.v.) solutions, pressure infusers and instruments for a cut-down.

• *Monitoring equipment:* transducers and a monitor capable of displaying two or three pressure waveforms, end-tidal carbon dioxide monitor and thermometer.

CRITERIA FOR DISCHARGE

Fully conscious and able to maintain their airway (although they may still be
 'sleepy')
Adequate breathing
Stable cardiovascular system, with minimal bleeding from the surgical site
Adequate pain relief
Warm

Table 7.1 Minimum criteria for discharge from recovery area.

DISCHARGE OF THE PATIENT

The anaesthetist's responsibility to the patient does not end with the termination of the anaesthetic. Although the care of the patient is handed
over to an appropriately trained and experienced recovery nurse (or
equivalent), the ultimate responsibility remains with the anaesthetist until
discharge from the recovery area. If there are inadequate recovery staff to
give appropriate care to a newly admitted patient then the anaesthetist
should continue to care for the patient.

> A patient who cannot maintain his/her own airway should never be
> left alone.

The length of time any patient spends in recovery will depend upon a
variety of factors, including: length and type of surgery, anaesthetic technique, and the occurrence of any complications. Most units have a policy
determining the minimum length of stay, which is usually around 30
minutes, and an agreed discharge criteria (Table 7.1).

Common complications and their management

The common complications seen in recovery are related to:
- the respiratory system;
- the cardiovascular system;
- nausea and vomiting.

THE RESPIRATORY SYSTEM

Hypoxaemia is the most important respiratory complication occurring
after anaesthesia and surgery. It occurs immediately on recovery and in
some patients for 3 or more days after surgery. It is traditionally recognized by the presence of cyanosis, but by this time the arterial Po_2 has

fallen to <8 kPa (55 mmHg), a saturation of 85%. The advent of the pulse oximeter has had a major impact on the early detection and prevention of hypoxaemia and should be used routinely in all patients. If hypoxaemia is severe or persistent, arterial blood gas analysis should be performed.

Causes of hypoxaemia

Hypoxaemia can be caused by a number of factors, either alone or in combination:

1 alveolar hypoventilation;
2 ventilation and perfusion mismatch within the lungs;
3 arteriovenous shunting of blood;
4 diffusion hypoxia;
5 pulmonary diffusion defects;
6 a reduced inspired oxygen concentration.

Alveolar hypoventilation

This is the commonest cause of hypoxaemia and can be due to a variety of causes (Table 7.2). On examination, a patient may exhibit signs of obstruction with abnormalities in rate, depth and effort of ventilation, asymmetry

---

CAUSES OF HYPOVENTILATION

Obstruction of the airway
The tongue
Blood, vomit, foreign bodies
Laryngeal spasm
Oedema or haematoma following surgery
Tumours

Central respiratory depression
Residual inhaled or i.v. general anaesthetic agents
Opioid analgesics
Hypocapnia
Hypothermia
An intracranial catastrophe

Impaired mechanics of ventilation
Pain
Residual neuromuscular blockade
Pneumothorax, haemothorax
Diaphragmatic splinting
Obesity

Table 7.2 Causes of hypoventilation.

of movement, and on auscultation, reduced breath sounds. Alveolar hypoventilation results in hypoxaemia because of insufficient influx of oxygen to replace that taken up by the blood, and as a result alveolar Po_2 (PAo_2) and arterial Po_2 (Pao_2) fall. In most cases, increasing the inspired oxygen concentration will restore alveolar and arterial Po_2. Ultimately, if ventilation is reduced further, no oxygen reaches the alveoli and profound hypoxaemia will follow irrespective of the inspired oxygen concentration. Despite the response to oxygen, the primary cause must also be identified and treated. Hypoventilation is always accompanied by hypercapnia as there is an inverse relationship between arterial carbon dioxide ($Paco_2$) and alveolar ventilation.

Obstruction of the airway

The *tongue* is the commonest cause, usually evidenced by noisy breathing. This is best prevented by recovering all patients in the lateral position, particularly those recovering from surgery where there is a risk of bleeding into the airway (e.g. ear, nose and throat (ENT) surgery), or regurgitation (bowel obstruction or a history of reflux). With increasing obstruction, breathing becomes quieter and more laboured until a stage is reached where the patient is making vigorous efforts, but with no ventilation. This produces a characteristic 'see-saw' or paradoxical pattern of ventilation. Diaphragmatic movement occurs as normal but there is indrawing of the ribs and intercostal muscles and a tracheal tug may be seen. Clearly, action must be taken urgently to relieve the obstruction.

If not already, turn the patient onto their left side (laryngoscopy is easier if subsequently required). If it is not possible to turn the patient (e.g. after a hip replacement), perform a chin lift or jaw thrust, both of which remove the tongue from the posterior wall of the pharynx (see page 188). An oropharyngeal or nasopharyngeal airway may be required to help maintain the airway (see page 39).

No patient should be handed to the care of the recovery nurse with noisy respiration of unknown cause.

Central respiratory depression

• *Residual effects of anaesthetic agents:* reduce the ventilatory response to hypoxia and hypercarbia and further contribute by reducing the level of consciousness.

• *Opioid analgesics:* may cause respiratory depression. Typically the patient has a low respiratory rate with a near normal tidal volume. The sedative effect of the drug may also reduce the level of consciousness. If severe, the administration of the specific antagonist naloxone may be required (see page 75).

• *Hypocapnia:* following excessive mechanical ventilation may reduce the drive to the respiratory centre and cause apnoea. This is usually only a problem where there is coexisting incomplete recovery from anaesthesia.

• *Hypothermia:* reduces ventilation but, in the absence of any contributing factors, it is usually adequate for the body's needs.

• *Intracranial catastrophe:* cerebral haemorrhage or ischaemia may cause direct damage to the respiratory centre or more commonly a deeply unconscious patient unable to maintain a patent airway.

Impaired mechanics of ventilation

• *Pain:* particularly after upper abdominal or thoracic surgery. Pain also prevents adequate coughing, leading to sputum retention and atelectasis, further impairing oxygenation.

• *Residual neuromuscular blockade:* seen as unsustained, jerky movements with rapid, shallow breathing. Such patients are often hypertensive and tachycardic due to the anxiety of being awake but partially paralysed! The diagnosis can be confirmed by using a nerve stimulator which is painful, or alternatively testing the ability to lift their head above the pillow for 5 seconds, or maintain a firm grip (see page 68). The ability to take a deep breath is not a very sensitive test. The patient should be given oxygen, reassured and sat upright to improve the efficiency of ventilation.

• *Pneumothorax or haemothorax:* prevents ventilation of the underlying lung.

• *Diaphragmatic splinting:* abdominal distension and obesity push the diaphragm into the thorax and increase the work of breathing. Such patients are greatly helped by being sat up which reduces the splinting of the diaphragm.

Ventilation and perfusion mismatch within the lungs

Normally, ventilation of the alveoli (V) and perfusion with blood (Q) are well matched ($V/Q = 1$) to ensure that the haemoglobin in blood leaving the lungs is saturated with oxygen. During anaesthesia, changes occur in the lungs which interfere with this process and these continue into the recovery period. This is referred to as ventilation perfusion (V/Q) mismatch. Areas develop where perfusion exceeds ventilation ($V/Q < 1$), resulting in haemoglobin with a reduced oxygen content. In other areas, ventilation exceeds perfusion ($V/Q > 1$), which can be considered wasted ventilation as very little additional oxygen is taken up as the haemoglobin is almost fully saturated. The net effect of this is that areas of overventilation cannot make up for the areas of overperfusion, and the result is a reduction in oxygen content of the blood leaving the lungs. All patients develop increased V/Q mismatch from the time of induction of general anaesthesia through to and including the recovery period. The aetiology of this is multifactorial but the following are recognized as being of major importance.

• *Mechanical ventilation:* causing a reduction in cardiac output will reduce perfusion of non-dependent areas of lung, whilst ventilation is maintained. This is worst in the lateral position, when the upper lung is better ventilated and the lower lung better perfused.

• *Reduced functional residual capacity (FRC):* in supine anaesthetized patients, particularly those over 50 years of age, this falls below their closing capacity — the lung volume below which some airways close and alveoli distal to this are no longer ventilated. Eventually, areas of atelectasis develop, mainly in dependent areas of the lung, leading to perfusion but no ventilation.

• *Pain:* particularly after abdominal surgery restricts breathing and coughing, leading to poor ventilation of the lung bases, sputum retention, basal atelectasis and ultimately infection. *This is worse in patients who smoke, are obese, have pre-existing lung disease, the elderly and after upper gastrointestinal or thoracic surgery, and is most prevalent at day three after surgery.*

Arteriovenous shunting of blood

True shunts are a result of a direct connection between the venous and arterial circulations causing hypoxaemia, for example in cyanotic congenital heart disease. The same shunting effect is seen in areas of the lung in which there is perfusion but no ventilation ($V/Q = 0$), as the blood remains deoxygenated, and is mixed with oxygenated blood leaving the lungs.

Normally, blood passing alveoli ventilated with air has an oxygen content of approximately 20 ml/100 ml blood. Shunted blood passing unventilated alveoli remains effectively venous, with an oxygen content of 15 ml/100 ml blood. Increasing the oxygen concentration in ventilated alveoli to 100% will only raise the oxygen content in blood passing these areas by 1 ml/100 ml blood to 21 ml/100 ml blood (Table 7.3). Therefore, for an equivalent blood flow, shunt has a more detrimental effect on oxygenation than breathing an increased oxygen concentration has on extra oxygen content. With small shunts, the hypoxaemia is correctable by increasing the inspired oxygen concentration, but by the time 30% of the blood flowing through the lungs is shunted, even 100% oxygen will have little effect on the arterial oxygenation due to the inability of the blood passing these areas to take up sufficient extra oxygen to offset the lack of oxygen in the shunted blood.

ALVEOLAR AND BLOOD OXYGEN CONTENT

Alveolar contents	Alveolar oxygen concentration (%)	Haemoglobin saturation (%)	Oxygen content (ml/100 ml blood)
Alveoli containing air	21	97	20
Alveoli containing oxygen	100	100	21
Non-ventilated alveoli	—	75	15

Table 7.3 Effect of alveolar oxygen concentration on oxygen content of blood.

Diffusion hypoxia
Nitrous oxide absorbed during anaesthesia has to be excreted. As it is very insoluble in blood, it rapidly diffuses down a concentration gradient into the alveoli, where it displaces oxygen. This reduces the partial pressure of oxygen in the alveoli, and renders the patient hypoxaemic. Arterial desaturation lasting several minutes may result. This is prevented by administering oxygen via a facemask (see below) to increase the inspired oxygen concentration.

Pulmonary diffusion defects
Any condition causing thickening of the alveolar membrane impairs transfer of oxygen into the blood, for example a pre-existing disease process such as fibrosing alveolitis. In the recovery period it may occur acutely, secondary to the development of pulmonary oedema as a result of fluid overload or impaired left ventricular function. The situation should be treated by first administering oxygen to increase the partial pressure of oxygen in the alveoli and then management of any underlying cause.

A reduced inspired oxygen concentration
As the inspired oxygen concentration is a prime determinant of the amount of oxygen in the alveoli, reducing this will lead to hypoxaemia. There are no circumstances where it is appropriate to administer less than 21% oxygen.

Management of hypoxaemia
All patients should be given oxygen for a number of reasons:
1 to counter the effects of diffusion hypoxia when nitrous oxide has been used;
2 to compensate for any hypoventilation;
3 to compensate for V/Q mismatch;
4 to meet the increased oxygen demands in patients who are shivering.

Patients who continue to hypoventilate, have persistent V/Q mismatch, are obese, anaemic or have ischaemic heart disease will require additional oxygen for an extended period of time. This is best determined either by arterial blood gas analysis or by using a pulse oximeter.

Devices used for delivery of oxygen

Variable-performance devices: masks or nasal cannulae

These are adequate for the majority of patients recovering from anaesthesia and surgery. The precise concentration of oxygen inspired by the patient is unknown as it is dependent upon the patient's respiratory pattern and the flow of oxygen used (usually 2–12 l/minute). The inspired gas consists of a mixture of:

- oxygen flowing into the mask;
- oxygen that has accumulated under the mask during the expiratory pause;
- alveolar gas containing carbon dioxide from the previous breath which has collected under the mask;
- air entrained during peak inspiratory flow from the holes in the side of the mask and from leaks between the mask and face.

Examples of this type of device are Hudson and MC masks (Fig. 7.1). As a guide, they increase the inspired oxygen concentration to 25–60% with oxygen flows 2–12 l/minute.

Some patients are unable to tolerate a facemask, and if they can nose

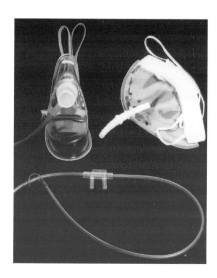

Fig. 7.1 Hudson mask (top left), MC mask (top right) and nasal catheters (bottom).

breathe either a single foam tipped catheter or double catheters can be used (see Fig. 7.1), placed just inside the vestibule of the nose. Lower flows of oxygen are used, 2–4 l/minute increasing the inspired oxygen concentration to 25–40%.

Fixed-performance devices

These are used when it is important to deliver a precise concentration of oxygen, unaffected by the patient's ventilatory pattern. These masks work on the principle of high airflow oxygen enrichment (HAFOE). Oxygen is fed into a venturi which entrains a much greater but constant flow of air, the total flow into the mask may be as high as 45 l/minute. Masks deliver either a fixed concentration or have interchangeable venturis to vary the oxygen concentration (Fig. 7.2). The high gas flow into the mask meets the patient's peak inspiratory flow—reducing entrainment of air—and flushes expiratory gas—reducing rebreathing.

If higher inspired oxygen concentrations are needed in a spontaneously breathing patient, a Hudson mask with a reservoir fitted can be used (see Fig. 7.2). A high flow of oxygen, 12–15 l/minute, is required, and the presence of a one-way valve ensures filling of the reservoir with oxygen during expiration, raising the concentration to 85%. An inspired oxygen concentration of 100% can only be achieved by using either an anaesthetic system with a close-fitting facemask or a self-inflating bag with reservoir and non-rebreathing valve and oxygen flow of 12–15 l/minute.

The above systems all deliver dry gas to the patient which causes crusting or thickening of secretions leading to difficulty with clearance.

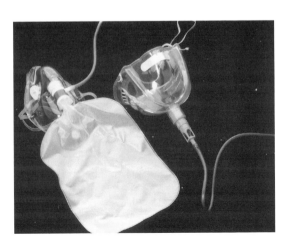

Fig. 7.2 Hudson mask with reservoir and high airflow oxygen enrichment (HAFOE; venturi) mask.

Gas from a HAFOE system should be passed through a humidifier for longer use.

THE CARDIOVASCULAR SYSTEM

Hypotension is the commonest cardiovascular complication arising in the postoperative period. It can be due to a variety of factors, alone or in combination:
* hypovolaemia;
* reduced myocardial contractility;
* vasodilatation;
* cardiac dysrhythmias.

Hypovolaemia

This is the commonest cause of hypotension after anaesthesia and surgery. The diagnosis can be confirmed by assessing the following:
* *Peripheral perfusion.* In the absence of fear, pain and hypothermia, cold clammy skin or delayed capillary refill (>2 seconds) suggests increased sympathetic activity secondary to hypovolaemia.
* *The radial pulse.* Note the rate and rhythm. A rapid pulse (>100 beats/minute) of poor volume suggests hypovolaemia.
* *Core and peripheral temperatures.* A low peripheral temperature in the presence of a normal core temperature is most often due to hypovolaemia with compensatory vasoconstriction.
* *Urine output.* Renal function is a sensitive indicator of cardiac output and tissue perfusion. Urine output is best measured hourly via a catheter and urometer. An inadequate urine output (<0.5 ml/kg per hour) may be due to:
  (a) a blocked catheter (blood clot or lubricant);
  (b) hypovolaemia;
  (c) hypotension;
  (d) hypoxia;
  (e) renal damage intraoperatively (e.g. during aneurysmal surgery).

> The commonest cause of oliguria is hypovolaemia; anuria is usually due to a blocked catheter.

* *Blood pressure.* In the presence of hypovolaemia, the systolic blood pressure is often initially near normal but the diastolic is elevated (narrow pulse pressure) as a result of compensatory vasoconstriction. The blood pressure must therefore always be interpreted in conjunction with the other assessments.

The extent to which these changes occur will depend primarily upon the degree of hypovolaemia. A tachycardia may not be seen in the patient taking β-blockers, the athlete may compensate with a heart rate well below 100 beats/minute and up to 15% of the blood volume may be lost without detectable signs in a fit, young patient.

If the facilities are available, an arterial blood sample should be analysed. A metabolic acidosis is usually found after a period of poor tissue perfusion. The trend of the patient's acid–base status is a useful indicator of therapeutic success.

Management
Although blood loss intraoperatively may be obvious, continued bleeding, especially in the absence of surgical drains may not be. It is important to inspect the surgical site for the development of any swelling and at the same time perform the following:
- Administer 100% oxygen via a facemask.
- Encourage venous return (head-down tilt or elevation of the legs).
- Administer i.v. fluids. Crystalloid or colloid 10–20 ml/kg body weight depending on the severity of the deficit. Blood loss of greater than 30% of the circulating volume will usually require the administration of cross-matched blood.
- Control external surgical bleeding by direct pressure, unless it is in the neck, compromising the airway when the wound should be decompressed (e.g. after thyroid surgery). Continued bleeding from any site requires surgical intervention.

Fluid loss may also occur as a result of tissue damage, leading to oedema or evaporation during prolonged surgery on body cavities, for example the abdomen or thorax (see below). Monitoring of the patient's central venous pressure (CVP) may be indicated if cardiac function is in question. In the presence of significant hypovolaemia *do not waste time inserting a CVP line for venous access alone.*

Reduced myocardial contractility

A frequent cause of this is ischaemic heart disease, in particular if there is any degree of left ventricular failure. At first this may present as evidence of poor peripheral circulation, a tachycardia and tachypnoea and can be difficult to distinguish from hypovolaemia. As the degree of ventricular failure worsens, the neck veins may become distended, the patient may become wheezy with a productive cough and on auscultation of the chest, a triple rhythm and basal crepitations are heard. A chest X-ray is usually diagnostic.

Management
- The patient should be sat upright.
- 100% oxygen is administered.
- The ECG, blood pressure and peripheral oxygen saturation should be monitored.

If the diagnosis is unclear, a fluid challenge (maximum 5 ml/kg) can be given and the response monitored, an improvement in the circulatory status indicating hypovolaemia. Where there is no doubt about the diagnosis, fluids can be restricted initially and a diuretic (e.g. frusemide 20–40 mg) given intravenously. Trends in the CVP can be monitored as a guide to therapy. If there is acute myocardial infarction, contractility may only improve with the use of inotropes in conjunction with vasodilators and this is best undertaken on the intensive care unit (ICU) (see page 166).

Vasodilatation

Any reduction in the systemic vascular resistance will cause hypotension (assuming the cardiac output is unchanged). Most commonly this is seen during spinal or epidural anaesthesia (see page 144). Blockade of the thoracolumbar segments of the spinal cord reduces sympathetic outflow to the vasculature, resulting in vasodilatation and hypotension. If the level of block extends above T5, there may be a bradycardia due to block of the cardiac sympathetic nerves. A similar effect is sometimes seen following prostate surgery under spinal anaesthesia. As the legs are taken down from the lithotomy position, the vascular compartment is suddenly extended and as the patient is moved to the recovery area, they become profoundly hypotensive.

Management
Hypotension secondary to regional anaesthesia is corrected by the administration of fluids (crystalloid, colloid, blood), the use of vasopressors (e.g. ephedrine), or a combination of both. The combination of hypovolaemia and vasodilatation result in profound hypotension. Oxygen should always be given.

Septic shock
Septic shock usually presents in the hours after the patient has left the recovery area, often during the night following daytime surgery. The initial presentation is peripheral vasodilatation, hypotension and tachycardia in the absence of blood loss. The patient may be pyrexial and if the cardiac output is measured, it is usually elevated. Gradually, vasoconstriction ensues along with a fall in cardiac output. The diagnosis should be

suspected in any patient who has had surgery associated with a septic focus, for example free infection in the peritoneal cavity or where there is infection in the genito-urinary tract. The causative microorganism is often a Gram-negative bacterium. These patients require early diagnosis, invasive monitoring and circulatory support on an ICU. Antibiotic therapy should be guided by a microbiologist.

Cardiac dysrhythmias

Dysrhythmias after anaesthesia are more common in the presence of hypoxaemia, hypercarbia, hypothermia, electrolyte abnormalities (hypokalaemia, hypocalcaemia), sepsis and pre-existing ischaemic heart disease. Correct management of these problems will result in spontaneous resolution of most dysrhythmias. Rarer causes include hypoadrenalism or hypothyroidism. Specific intervention is required if there is a significant reduction in cardiac output and hypotension. Bradycardias can reduce the heart rate below the point where no further increase in stroke volume can take place to maintain cardiac output, whereas tachycardias result in insufficient time for ventricular filling, and stroke volume and cardiac output fall.

> Coronary artery flow is dependent on diastolic pressure and time. Hypotension and tachycardia are therefore particularly dangerous.

Sinus tachycardia (> 100 beats/minute)

This is the commonest dysrhythmia after anaesthesia and surgery, usually as a result of pain or alternatively hypovolaemia due to inadequate fluid administration intraoperatively or postoperatively. Occasionally, if associated with a pyrexia, it may be an early indication of sepsis.

Treatment consists of oxygen, analgesia and adequate fluid replacement. If the tachycardia persists, then *providing there is no contraindication*, a small dose of a β-blocker may be given intravenously whilst monitoring the ECG. Rarely, the development of an unexplained tachycardia after anaesthesia may be the first sign of malignant hyperpyrexia (see page 69).

Supraventricular tachycardias

The most common of these is probably rapid atrial fibrillation (> 130 beats/minute). Expert help should be sought and if symptomatic, early cardioversion will probably be required. In the stable patient, pharmacological management can be used, again under the guidance of an expert.

Sinus bradycardia (<60 beats/minute)

This may be seen:
• following the reversal of neuromuscular block when an inadequate dose of either atropine or glycopyrrolate is administered with neostigmine;
• during the use of suction to clear pharyngeal or tracheal secretions;
• in association with the development of acute inferior myocardial infarction;
• in patients taking β-blockers preoperatively (or if administered intraoperatively).

Treatment should consist of removing any provoking stimuli and administering oxygen. If symptomatic, atropine 0.5 mg intravenously may be required.

Hypertension

This is often the result of pain, hypoxaemia or hypercarbia and is more likely to be of greater severity in patients with pre-existing hypertension. A coexisting tachycardia is particularly dangerous in the presence of ischaemic heart disease as this may cause an acute myocardial infarction. If the blood pressure remains elevated after correcting the above, a vasodilator or β-blocker may be necessary.

NAUSEA AND VOMITING

This occurs in up to 80% of patients following anaesthesia and surgery. A variety of factors have been identified which increase the incidence.
• Age and sex: more common in young women and children.
• Site of surgery: abdominal, middle ear or the posterior cranial fossa.
• Administration of opioid analgesics pre-, intra- and postoperatively.
• Anaesthetic drugs: etomidate, nitrous oxide.
• Gastric dilatation, caused by manual ventilation with a bag and mask without a clear airway.
• Hypotension associated with epidural or spinal anaesthesia.
• Patients prone to travel sickness.

Drugs used to treat nausea and vomiting

Before resorting to the administration of drugs to treat nausea and vomiting, it is essential to make sure that the patient is not hypoxaemic or hypotensive.
• *Phenothiazine derivatives:* prochlorperazine (Stemetil). Adults 12.5 mg intramuscularly 6-hourly or 15–30 mg orally, daily in divided doses. May cause hypotension due to α-blockade. Some have antihistamine activity and may cause dystonic muscle movements.

- *Dopamine antagonists:* metoclopramide (Maxolon). Adults 10 mg intravenously, intramuscularly or orally, 6-hourly. A specific anti-emetic, not related to the major tranquillizers and has no sedative or antihistamine effects. Has an effect at the chemoreceptor trigger zone and increases gastric motility. An alternative is domperidone (Motilium) 10 mg orally.
- *5-HT3 (hydroxytryptamine) antagonists:* ondansetron (Zofran). Adults 4–8 mg intravenously or orally, 8-hourly. Has both central and peripheral actions. In the gut it blocks 5-HT3 receptors in the mucosal vagal afferents. It does not cause dystonic movements.
- *Antihistamines:* cyclizine. Adults 50 mg intramuscularly. Also has anticholinergic actions. A combined preparation with morphine (Cyclimorph) is available.
- *Butyrophenone derivatives:* droperidol (Droleptan). Adults 1.5 mg intravenously. Larger doses have no increased anti-emetic action. Effective at the chemoreceptor trigger zone. May cause extrapyramidal side-effects.

The anticholinergic agents, atropine and hyoscine both have mild anti-emetic actions.

MISCELLANEOUS COMPLICATIONS AFTER ANAESTHESIA

- *Haematoma:* may develop on removal of a cannula or at a site where cannulation was unsuccessful. Thrombophlebitis may occur after prolonged cannulation for an i.v. infusion (>12 hours) causing pain for several weeks.
- *Intubation:* may cause trauma to the lips, teeth, pharynx, larynx (and nose during nasal intubation). A sore throat is common, but may also have been caused by the insertion of a nasogastric tube or the use of an oropharyngeal airway. Persistent hoarseness may indicate the development of a laryngeal granuloma, necessitating referral to an ENT surgeon.
- *Suxamethonium:* may be followed by muscle pains postoperatively, most commonly in young, physically fit women who are ambulant soon after recovery. The muscles of the neck, shoulders and upper thorax are most affected. It resolves spontaneously after a few days.
- *Headaches:* common, but a specific cause following general anaesthesia has not been identified. It is a well-recognized complication of spinal anaesthesia (see page 145).
- *Retention of urine:* more likely to occur when there is a pre-existing history of prostatism. Spinal and epidural anaesthesia remove the sensation of bladder fullness. Excretion of the fluid load used to maintain the blood pressure may lead to overstretching of the bladder, impairing the ability to urinate when sensation returns. Pathological causes must always

be considered when a patient fails to pass urine postoperatively, for example a period of intraoperative hypotension or hypoxia, or pre-existing renal disease. Surgery may have inadvertently interfered with either the renal blood supply or damaged the ureters. If catheterization is required, it must be performed aseptically, and depending upon the type of surgery that has been performed, prophylactic antibiotics may be required.

Postoperative analgesia

Inadequate analgesia is a contributing factor in all the common postoperative complications. Ignorance, and fear of respiratory depression and addiction has lead to woefully inadequate postoperative pain relief for many patients. Until recently it was not uncommon to find a fixed dose of an analgesic (e.g. morphine) being administered intramuscularly when the patient requested it, providing this was not more frequent than 4-hourly! This is clearly inadequate, the absorption, distribution, metabolism and effect of opioids varies greatly and in surgical patients the plasma levels of morphine required for adequate analgesia can vary up to eightfold. Many factors are recognized as influencing the severity of postoperative pain and analgesic requirement.

- *Site of operation*. Upper abdominal and thoracic surgery causes the most severe pain of the longest duration, control of which is important because of the detrimental effects on ventilation. Pain caused by surgery to the body wall or periphery of limbs is less severe and for a shorter duration.
- *Psychological factors*. Frightened, anxious patients require more analgesics than those who are well prepared and calm, due partly to an increased perception of pain. The preoperative visit by the anaesthetist plays a significant role in allaying fears and anxiety.
- *Age and sex*. Older patients tend to require lower doses of analgesics as a result of changes in drug distribution and coexisting disease. Prescribing should take account of this rather than being used as an excuse for inadequate analgesia. There is no difference in the amount of pain suffered by different sexes having the same operation.
- *Anaesthetic management*. The use of analgesic drugs intraoperatively, or the use of regional anaesthesia, will influence the severity of pain on recovery and the need for analgesia.
- *Body weight*. This has minimal influence on the amount of a drug which needs to be given to achieve effective analgesia. However, it does affect the amount of drug which needs to be given to achieve a therapeutic blood level. Drug elimination (usually dependent on renal or hepatic function)

determines the rate at which a drug must be given to achieve steady state and, therefore, continuing analgesia.

RELIEF OF POSTOPERATIVE PAIN

The use of intermittent intramuscular (i.m.) injections for pain relief post-operatively is made more effective by:
• prescribing a range of doses which may be administered, for example 5–10 mg morphine;
• reducing the time limit between doses to 1 hour;
• frequently assessing and quantifying the severity of the patient's pain, level of sedation and any complications (see below):

1 *Severity of pain.* Several methods are used. One method is to use a linear analogue scale consisting of a 10 cm line, at one end is marked zero (no pain) and at the other end is marked 10 (the worst pain imaginable). The patient marks the line to indicate the severity of their pain. A more simple alternative is a description of severity which can be scaled for recording:

0 = no pain;
1 = mild pain;
2 = moderate pain;
3 = severe pain.

In the absence of any contraindications, moderate and severe pain (scores of 2–3) indicate the need for analgesia.

2 *Sedation.* This can be assessed and scored using the following four-point scale:

0 = no sedation, patient alert;
1 = mild sedation, occasionally drowsy, easy to rouse;
2 = moderately sedated, frequently drowsy, easy to rouse;
3 = severely sedated, somnolent, difficult to rouse.

Figure 7.3 shows an algorithm for improving the effectiveness of i.m. administration of morphine.

Points to note

• *Onset of analgesia after i.m. administration can often be delayed.* This can be overcome by giving the first dose intravenously. The opioid used should be diluted (e.g. 10 mg morphine or 100 mg pethidine in 10 ml saline) and given in 1–2 ml increments every 5–10 minutes until the desired effect is achieved.
• *Consider the use of pethidine for:*
   (a) asthmatic patients, as it causes less histamine release than morphine;
   (b) patients after biliary surgery and those who have had bowel ana-stomoses, as it has less effect on smooth muscle.

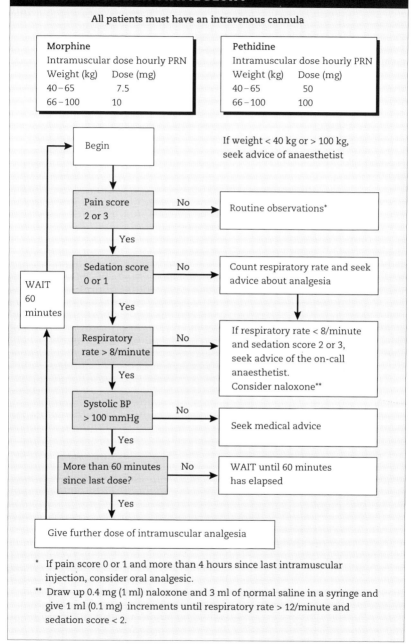

ALGORITHM FOR POSTOPERATIVE INTRAMUSCULAR ANALGESIA

All patients must have an intravenous cannula

Morphine	
Intramuscular dose hourly PRN	
Weight (kg)	Dose (mg)
40–65	7.5
66–100	10

Pethidine	
Intramuscular dose hourly PRN	
Weight (kg)	Dose (mg)
40–65	50
66–100	100

Begin

If weight < 40 kg or > 100 kg, seek advice of anaesthetist

Pain score 2 or 3 — No → Routine observations*

Yes

Sedation score 0 or 1 — No → Count respiratory rate and seek advice about analgesia

Yes

WAIT 60 minutes

Respiratory rate > 8/minute — No → If respiratory rate < 8/minute and sedation score 2 or 3, seek advice of the on-call anaesthetist. Consider naloxone**

Yes

Systolic BP > 100 mmHg — No → Seek medical advice

Yes

More than 60 minutes since last dose? — No → WAIT until 60 minutes has elapsed

Yes

Give further dose of intramuscular analgesia

* If pain score 0 or 1 and more than 4 hours since last intramuscular injection, consider oral analgesic.

** Draw up 0.4 mg (1 ml) naloxone and 3 ml of normal saline in a syringe and give 1 ml (0.1 mg) increments until respiratory rate > 12/minute and sedation score < 2.

Fig. 7.3 Algorithm for postoperative intramuscular analgesia. After Gould TH *et al*. Policy for controlling pain after surgery. *British Medical Journal* 1992; **305**: 1187–93.

- *Non-steroidal anti-inflammatory drugs (NSAIDs):* may be sufficient after minor surgery and may be used in conjunction with opioids to reduce the dose, and potential, for side-effects. Ketorolac can be given intravenously or intramuscularly, an initial dose of 10 mg, followed by 10–30 mg 4- to 6-hourly up to a maximum of 90 mg/day (60 mg/day for the elderly) for 2 days.
- *Following minor peripheral surgery:* patients may only need oral analgesia. Compound preparations of paracetamol with codeine phosphate are frequently effective, for example paracetamol 500 mg plus codeine phosphate 30 mg, 1–2 tablets 4- to 6-hourly, up to a maximum of eight per day.

In many units, control of postoperative pain by i.m. injections has been surpassed by using the following techniques.

PATIENT-CONTROLLED ANALGESIA

Patient-controlled analgesia (PCA) consists of a microprocessor-controlled syringe pump capable of being programmed to deliver a predetermined bolus dose of a drug intravenously. Activation is by the patient depressing a switch which is designed to prevent accidental triggering (hence 'patient-controlled'). In addition, there may be a background low-dose continuous infusion. Three safety measures exist to prevent the administration of an overdose:

1 the bolus dose and any background infusion is preset (usually by a doctor);

2 after successful administration of a bolus dose, a subsequent dose cannot be administered for a preset period, termed the 'lockout period';

3 the total quantity of drug administered over a predetermined period can be limited.

Typical settings for an adult using morphine delivered by a PCA device might be:

bolus dose: 1 mg;

lockout interval: 6 minutes;

4-hourly dose limit: 30 mg.

In order for PCA to be used effectively the following principles must be observed.

- Preoperatively, the patient must be briefed by the anaesthetist and/or nursing staff and if possible, shown the device to be used.
- Before commencing PCA, a loading dose of analgesic should be given, usually intravenously. Failure to do this will result in the patient being unable to get sufficient analgesia from the PCA device and the system will fail.

PCA OVERDOSE MANAGEMENT

- Stop the PCA
- Give oxygen via a mask
- Call for assistance
- Consider giving naloxone (as described for intramuscular opioids)
- If the patient is apnoeic, commence ventilation using a self-inflating bag-valve-mask device

Table 7.4 Management of overdose with patient-controlled analgesia (PCA).

- A dedicated i.v. cannula or non-return valve on an i.v. infusion must be used to prevent accumulation of the drug and failure of analgesia.
- The patient's pain score, sedation score and respiratory rate must be observed and recorded to ensure success.
- If on any assessment, or at any other time, the respiratory rate is less than 8 beats/minute and the sedation score is 2 or 3, treat the patient as described in Table 7.4.

Advantages

- Greater flexibility, and matching of analgesic administration to the patient's perception of the pain.
- Reduced workload for the nursing staff.
- Elimination of painful i.m. injections.
- Intravenous administration with greater certainty of adequate plasma levels.

Disadvantages

- The equipment is initially expensive to purchase and there are ongoing costs of syringes and appropriate tubing for administration.
- The patient must understand what is required and be physically able to trigger the device.
- There is always the potential for overdose if the device is incorrectly programmed.

As pain subsides the PCA can be discontinued, and oral analgesics can be used. The first dose should be given 1 hour prior to discontinuing PCA, to ensure continuity of analgesia. An algorithm for PCA is given in Fig. 7.4.

INTRAVENOUS INFUSIONS OF OPIOID ANALGESICS

In this technique, a continuous i.v. infusion of an opioid drug is given from a syringe pump, the rate of which can be varied. The drug is administered

ALGORITHM FOR PATIENT-CONTROLLED ANALGESIA

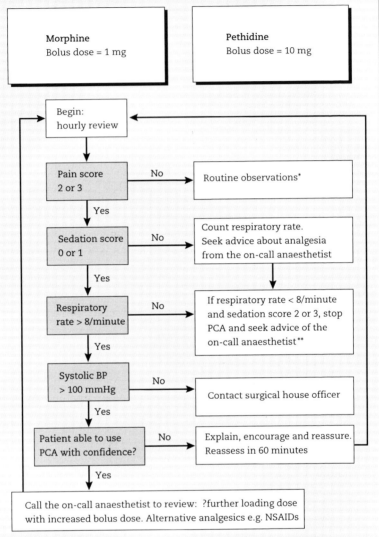

Morphine	Pethidine
Bolus dose = 1 mg	Bolus dose = 10 mg

Begin: hourly review

Pain score 2 or 3 → No → Routine observations*

↓ Yes

Sedation score 0 or 1 → No → Count respiratory rate. Seek advice about analgesia from the on-call anaesthetist

↓ Yes

Respiratory rate > 8/minute → No → If respiratory rate < 8/minute and sedation score 2 or 3, stop PCA and seek advice of the on-call anaesthetist**

↓ Yes

Systolic BP > 100 mmHg → No → Contact surgical house officer

↓ Yes

Patient able to use PCA with confidence? → No → Explain, encourage and reassure. Reassess in 60 minutes

↓ Yes

Call the on-call anaesthetist to review: ?further loading dose with increased bolus dose. Alternative analgesics e.g. NSAIDs

* If pain score 0 or 1 and tolerating oral intake, consider oral analgesic.

** If patient apnoeic, use bag and mask to ventilate. Draw up 0.4 mg (1 ml) naloxone and 3 ml of normal saline in a syringe. Give 1 ml (0.1 mg) increments until respiratory rate > 12/minute and sedation score < 2.

Fig. 7.4 Algorithm for patient-controlled analgesia (PCA). After Gould TH et al. Policy for controlling pain after surgery. *British Medical Journal* 1992; **305**: 1187–93.

into a dedicated i.v. cannula following a loading dose as for PCA. A typical starting rate for an infusion of morphine in a young, fit patient with normal renal and hepatic function is between 3 and 5 mg/hour. A frail, older patient may only require 1 mg/hour. Regular assessment as for PCA is required and the rate of infusion adjusted within the predetermined limits to maintain analgesia. Older syringe pumps are set to deliver volume (usually in ml/hour) and therefore the concentration of drug used must be clearly identified. Often a dilution of 1 mg/ml is used. Ideally, this technique is best suited to use in patients on either a high dependency unit or ICU.

Points to note

• *Pain due to an inadequate rate of infusion:* can be rectified by a doctor or qualified nurse giving small incremental bolus doses to effect and then increasing the infusion rate. Simply increasing the infusion rate is inadequate because it will take hours for the plasma drug level to rise appreciably.

• *If the infusion rate is too high:* in addition to profound analgesia the patient will become increasingly drowsy, with evidence of respiratory depression (less than 8 breaths/minute). Proceed as described for PCA overdose (see Table 7.4).

Advantages

• Avoids large swings in pain control by achieving steady state plasma levels, particularly while the patient is asleep.

• Ultimately saves nursing staff time.

• It is an ideal method for providing analgesia in ventilated patients who are incapable of demanding pain control.

• It is useful in patients who are physically unable to manage a PCA device, for example those with severe rheumatoid disease.

Disadvantages

• Blood levels of morphine will accumulate if the rate of elimination is less than that of the infusion. Patients should therefore be closely monitored. For this reason it is not wise to use this technique on the open ward.

• The correct infusion rate to maintain adequate analgesia can only be achieved after trial and error, which requires a period of intense input from a physician or nurse trained in its use.

Total drug consumption per 24 hours

The total amount of drug consumed per 24 hours can be calculated to allow the patient's progress to be monitored and indirectly checks that the equipment is performing as desired. This is particularly important when pethidine is used because the metabolites may cause seizures when more than 1200 mg are infused in an adult over a 24-hour period.

Record keeping and audit

Patients using PCA or infusion devices should be reviewed daily by a suitably trained person (e.g. a nurse, doctor or pharmacist) and adjustments made to the settings of the equipment used according to the patient's needs aided by the charted information.

An algorithm for infusion analgesia is given in Fig. 7.5.

EPIDURAL (EXTRADURAL) ANALGESIA FOR POSTOPERATIVE PAIN CONTROL

Infusions of a local anaesthetic, either alone or in combination with opioids into the epidural space provide dramatic relief of postoperative pain following major surgery. Originally used in intensive care or high dependency units, this technique is becoming increasingly popular for patients nursed on the ward postoperatively. It is essential that patients are counselled by the anaesthetist and nursing staff on the ward before surgery and warned of altered sensation and potential weakness of the lower limbs postoperatively.

Catheter placement

The epidural is most often established by the anaesthetist preoperatively and used as part of the anaesthetic technique. For upper abdominal surgery an epidural in the mid-thoracic region (T6/7) is used while a hip operation would need a lumbar epidural (L1/2).

Many different combinations of local anaesthetic and opioid have been used successfully. Ideally, the concentration of local anaesthetic should block sensory nerves, leaving motor nerves relatively spared. The choice and dose of opioid should be such that the drug passes through the dura into the cerebrospinal fluid (CSF) in sufficient quantities to block the opioid receptors in the spinal cord but does not spread cranially to cause respiratory depression. Examples of such combinations are bupivacaine 0.167% plus diamorphine 0.1 mg/ml, and bupivacaine 0.125% plus fentanyl 4 µg/ml. These are often prepared under sterile conditions by the pharmacy department to reduce the risk of errors and contamination. In patients over the age of 60 years, the amount of opioid is often halved.

The infusion rate and the site of the catheter determine the spread of the solution, being greatest in the thoracic epidural space where a starting infusion rate might be 4 ml/hour. In the lumbar space it is reasonable to commence a higher infusion rate, for example 8 ml/hour. Once started,

ALGORITHM FOR POSTOPERATIVE INFUSION ANALGESIA

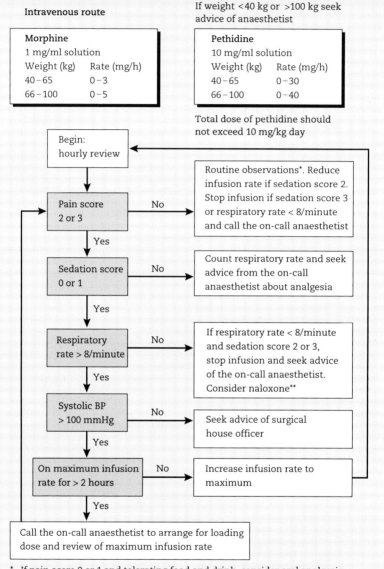

Intravenous route

If weight <40 kg or >100 kg seek advice of anaesthetist

Morphine 1 mg/ml solution	
Weight (kg)	Rate (mg/h)
40–65	0–3
66–100	0–5

Pethidine 10 mg/ml solution	
Weight (kg)	Rate (mg/h)
40–65	0–30
66–100	0–40

Total dose of pethidine should not exceed 10 mg/kg day

Begin: hourly review

Pain score 2 or 3 → No → Routine observations*. Reduce infusion rate if sedation score 2. Stop infusion if sedation score 3 or respiratory rate < 8/minute and call the on-call anaesthetist

↓ Yes

Sedation score 0 or 1 → No → Count respiratory rate and seek advice from the on-call anaesthetist about analgesia

↓ Yes

Respiratory rate > 8/minute → No → If respiratory rate < 8/minute and sedation score 2 or 3, stop infusion and seek advice of the on-call anaesthetist. Consider naloxone**

↓ Yes

Systolic BP > 100 mmHg → No → Seek advice of surgical house officer

↓ Yes

On maximum infusion rate for > 2 hours → No → Increase infusion rate to maximum

↓ Yes

Call the on-call anaesthetist to arrange for loading dose and review of maximum infusion rate

* If pain score 0 or 1 and tolerating food and drink, consider oral analgesic.
** Draw up 0.4 mg (1 ml) naloxone and 3 ml of normal saline in a syringe and give 1 ml (0.1 mg) increments until respiratory rate > 12/minute and sedation score < 2.

Fig. 7.5 Algorithm for infusion analgesia. After Gould TH *et al.* Policy for controlling pain after surgery. *British Medical Journal* 1992; **305**: 1187–93.

the efficacy of the infusion must be monitored in a similar manner as for PCA. If analgesia proves inadequate, then it may become necessary to administer a bolus dose. Observations of the patients vital signs should then be made on a regular basis according to local protocol.

Complications arising during epidural analgesia

This will depend upon whether local anaesthetics alone or in combination with opioids have been used. The complications arising as a result of the use of local anaesthetics are covered on page 136.

• *Sedation:* usually due to the opioid reaching the brain either directly via the CSF or after absorption into the systemic circulation via the epidural veins. It may eventually lead to respiratory depression and unconsciousness (see below). Occasionally, sedation may be secondary to hypotension and cerebral hypoxaemia. The infusion should be stopped and the patient's vital signs assessed. If the patient is unresponsive, or the level of sedation progresses, it can be reversed by giving naloxone in 0.1 mg increments intravenously and expert help should be sought.

• *Respiratory depression:* caused by opioid reaching the respiratory centre in the medulla. Highly lipid soluble opioids, for example diamorphine, are rapidly taken up by the spinal cord, limiting their spread and systemic absorption and respiratory depression tends to occur early. Less soluble opioids, for example morphine, are taken up slowly, and respiratory depression tends to occur later. A high infusion rate of either drug may also lead to respiratory depression. Treatment consists initially of stopping the epidural infusion, supporting the ventilation if necessary, and administering naloxone, according to the severity. Expert help should be sought.

• *Pruritus:* this can sometimes be troublesome and is frequently localized to the nose. It may respond to antihistamines, atropine or naloxone.

• *Retention of urine:* urine output should be monitored routinely in all postoperative patients. When an epidural is used for pain relief, failure to pass urine may be due to the effect of the opioid on bladder sphincter control or the local anaesthetic removing the sensation of a full bladder. It should be managed as described on page 118.

An algorithm for epidural infusion analgesia is given in Fig. 7.6.

Postoperative intravenous fluid therapy

Not all patients require routine i.v. fluids after anaesthesia and surgery. For those that do, the volume and type of fluid will be determined by a variety of factors including:

ALGORITHM FOR EPIDURAL INFUSION ANALGESIA

Bupivacaine: 0.167%	60 ml (syringe pump) = 20 ml 0.5% + 40 ml normal saline
Diamorphine:	
0 mg/ml	0 mg
(> 60 years) 0.05 mg/ml	3 mg
0.1 mg/ml	6 mg

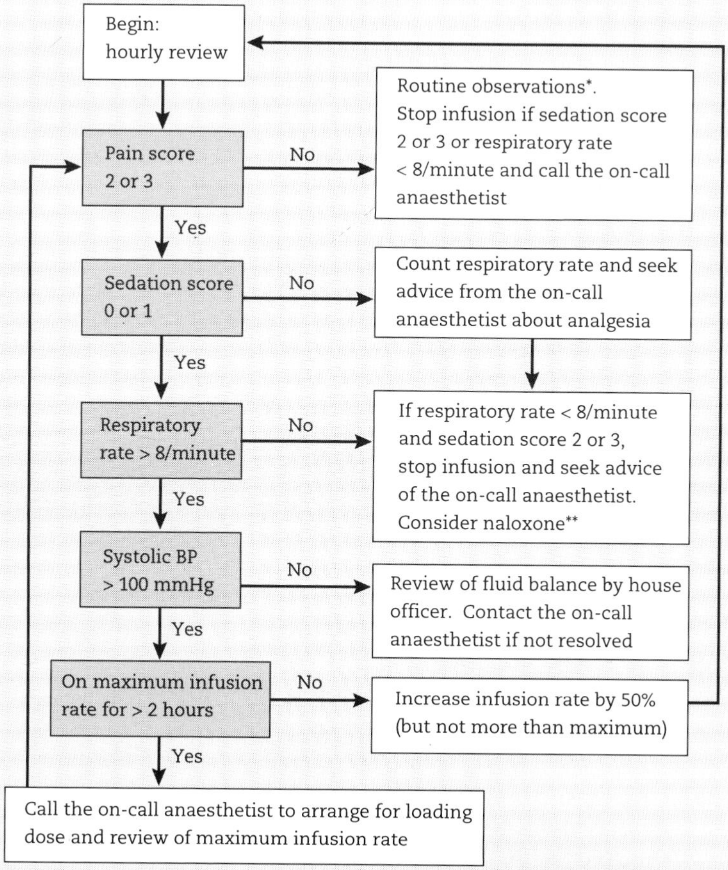

Begin: hourly review

Pain score 2 or 3 — **No** → Routine observations*. Stop infusion if sedation score 2 or 3 or respiratory rate < 8/minute and call the on-call anaesthetist

Yes ↓

Sedation score 0 or 1 — **No** → Count respiratory rate and seek advice from the on-call anaesthetist about analgesia

Yes ↓

Respiratory rate > 8/minute — **No** → If respiratory rate < 8/minute and sedation score 2 or 3, stop infusion and seek advice of the on-call anaesthetist. Consider naloxone**

Yes ↓

Systolic BP > 100 mmHg — **No** → Review of fluid balance by house officer. Contact the on-call anaesthetist if not resolved

Yes ↓

On maximum infusion rate for > 2 hours — **No** → Increase infusion rate by 50% (but not more than maximum)

Yes ↓

Call the on-call anaesthetist to arrange for loading dose and review of maximum infusion rate

* If pain score 1 and tolerating fluids, consider oral analgesic.
** Draw up 0.4 mg (1 ml) naloxone and 3 ml of normal saline in a syringe and give 1 ml (0.1 mg) increments until respiratory rate > 12/minute and sedation score < 2.

Fig. 7.6 Algorithm for epidural analgesia. After Gould TH *et al.* Policy for controlling pain after surgery. *British Medical Journal* 1992; **305**: 1187–93.

- any delay in starting to drink;
- the site of surgery;
- the extent of tissue damage;
- blood loss during and after surgery;
- continuing losses from the gastrointestinal tract.

A wide range of fluids are available (see page 99) and for each patient the type and volume will be dependent upon the calculated maintenance requirements of water and electrolytes plus the replacement of any abnormal losses. This is complemented by clinical evaluation of the patient to ensure that they are adequately hydrated, as assessed by degree of thirst, moisture of mucous membranes, blood pressure, pulse, peripheral circulation and an adequate urine output. In complex cases, monitoring the trend of the CVP may also prove useful.

MINOR SURGERY

Following minor surgical procedures (i.e. taking less than 30 minutes, with minimal blood loss and tissue trauma), i.v. fluids are not required as most patients start drinking within 1–2 hours of surgery. However, if the patient has failed to drink within 4–6 hours (usually as a result of nausea and vomiting) then consideration should be given to commencing i.v. fluids. Providing that the volume of vomit is not excessive, then only maintenance fluids are required, calculated at 1.5 ml/kg per hour, the volume of which must take into account the accrued deficit. For example, a 70 kg patient starved from 0800 to 1400, who is still unable to take fluids by mouth at 1800 will require:

1.5 ml/kg per hour to make up the deficit from 0800 until 1800

$$= 1.5 \times 70 \ (kg) \times 10 \ (hour) \approx 1000 \, ml;$$

1.5 ml/kg per hour from 1800 until 0800 the next morning

$$= 1.5 \times 70 \ (kg) \times 14 \ (hour) \approx 1400 \, ml.$$

The total i.v. fluid requirement = 2400 ml in the next 14 hours. This should contain the daily requirement of Na^+ (1 mmol/kg) = 70 mmol. An appropriate prescription would therefore be:

- 1000 ml over the first 4 hours;
- 1000 ml over the following 6 hours;
- 500 ml over the last 4 hours.
  This could be given either as:
- 2 × 1000 ml 5% glucose and 500 ml 0.9% (normal) saline; or
- 2 × 1000 ml 4% glucose/0.18% saline, and 500 ml 4% glucose/0.18% saline.

This should then be reviewed at 0800 with regard to further management.

MAJOR SURGERY

Following major surgery, postoperative fluid balance is more complex. Assuming that appropriate volumes of water, electrolytes and blood have been given during the operation, then postoperatively the fluid and electrolyte requirements will depend upon:

- the volume needed for ongoing maintenance, which will be increased if the patient is pyrexial;
- the replacement of continuing losses from the gastrointestinal tract, for example via a nasogastric tube;
- any continued bleeding;
- rewarming of cold peripheries causing vasodilatation.

The patient who has undergone major surgery will require close monitoring to ensure that sufficient volumes of the correct fluid are administered. A standard postoperative regimen for the first 24 hours postoperatively might therefore consist of:

- 1.5 ml/kg per hour water, increased by 10% for each °C if the patient is pyrexial;
- sodium, 1 mmol/kg;
- replacement of measured gastrointestinal losses with an equal volume of Hartmann's solution;
- replacement of blood loss of < 500 ml with either:
  (a) Hartmann's solution (remember, three times the volume of blood lost will be needed as it is distributed throughout the extracellular fluid (ECF)); or
  (b) colloid, the same volume as the blood loss;
- replacement of blood loss > 1000 ml with stored blood.

On the second and subsequent days, the same basic principles are used. In addition, potassium is required (in addition to sodium) at the rate of 1 mmol/kg per 24 hours. Precise adjustment of the amount of electrolytes needed is guided by reference to the previous day's serum electrolytes.

If surgery has been associated with significant tissue trauma (e.g. total hip replacement, aortic aneurysm surgery), then there will be continued losses into the tissues, which has the same effect as any other form of fluid loss and is often referred to as 'third space losses'. Such volumes are difficult to measure and usually become evident as a result of the above regimen failing to keep the patient adequately hydrated. This is usually seen as thirst, a dry mouth, cool peripheries with empty superficial veins, hypotension, tachycardia and a decrease in the urine output to less than

0.5 ml/kg per hour. An additional 1 l of Hartmann's solution may need to be added to the above regimen to account for such losses and adjusted according to the patient's response. These losses may continue for up to 48 hours after surgery and sufficient extra volumes of fluid should be administered to maintain hydration and an adequate circulating volume. Where large volumes of fluid are required and/or there is underlying heart disease, then the CVP should be measured and the trend noted (see page 82) and serum electrolytes monitored twice daily.

The stress response

Following major surgery and trauma, various neuroendocrine responses result in an increased secretion of a variety of hormones. Antidiuretic hormone (ADH) secretion is maximal during surgery and may remain elevated for several days. The effect of this is to increase water absorption by the kidneys and reduce urine output. Aldosterone secretion is raised secondary to increased cortisol levels and activation of the renin-angiotensin system. This results in sodium retention and increased urinary excretion of potassium. Despite this retention of water and sodium, it is important that fluid input is not restricted in these patients, as the continued losses identified above more than offset the volume retained.

After 2–3 days, hormone levels return to normal and this is followed by an increase in the volume of urine passed, which may be augmented by loss of fluid as tissue oedema resolves.

Further reading

Bay I, Nunn JF, Prys Roberts C. Factors affecting arterial PO_2 during recovery from general anaesthesia. *British Journal of Anaesthesia* 1968; **40**: 398–407.

Moote CA. The prevention of postoperative pain. *Canadian Journal of Anaesthesia* 1994; **41**: 527–33.

Shelly MP, Eltringham RJ. Rational fluid therapy during surgery. *British Journal of Hospital Medicine* 1988; **39**: 506–17.

Watcha MF, White PF. Postoperative nausea and vomiting. Its etiology, treatment and prevention. *Anesthesiology* 1992; **77**: 162–84.

West JB. *Respiratory Physiology — the Essentials*, 5th edn. Baltimore: Williams and Wilkins, 1994.

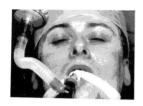

Local and Regional Anaesthesia

When referring to local and regional techniques and the drugs used, the terms 'analgesia' and 'anaesthesia' are used very loosely and interchangeably. For clarity and consistency the following terms will be used:
• *Analgesia:* the state when only relief of pain is provided. This may allow some minor surgical procedures to be performed, for example infiltration analgesia for suturing.
• *Anaesthesia:* the state when analgesia is accompanied by muscle relaxation, usually to allow major surgery to be undertaken. Regional anaesthesia may be used alone or in combination with general anaesthesia.

All drugs will be referred to as local anaesthetics irrespective of the technique for which they are being used.

Pharmacology of local anaesthetic agents

Local anaesthetics can be divided into two groups on the basis of their chemical structure.
1 *Amides:* lignocaine, prilocaine and bupivacaine.
2 *Esters:* amethocaine, benzocaine, procaine and cocaine.

The esters were the first agents to be introduced into clinical practice. However, they are relatively more toxic, allergenic and less stable than their modern counterparts, the amides. They are still occasionally used topically for surface anaesthesia (e.g. amethocaine lozenges for the oropharynx and cocaine for nasal surgery). All amide local anaesthetics are metabolized in the liver by enzymes (amidases). In patients with reduced liver function, reduced doses must be used, for example in the elderly, frail or shocked.

Lignocaine (Xylocaine)

This is a versatile agent which can be used for infiltration, nerve blocks,

133

intravenous regional analgesia (IVRA) and epidural and spinal anaesthesia. It is available in many concentrations (0.5–10%), with or without adrenaline. It has a relatively fast onset and a duration of action of 60–180 minutes, depending upon the technique used. It is a mild vasodilator. The currently accepted maximum safe dose of lignocaine is:

- 3 mg/kg, maximum 200 mg (without adrenaline);
- 6 mg/kg, maximum 500 mg (with adrenaline).

Prilocaine (Citanest)

Closely related to lignocaine and equipotent, it is used mainly for infiltration, nerve blocks and IVRA. It is supplied in 0.5–2% solutions plus or minus adrenaline. Speed of onset is similar to lignocaine but duration of action is slightly longer. There is no vasodilatation, absorption is slower and it is less toxic, as a result of which it is now the agent of choice for IVRA (Bier's block). In overdose, a metabolite (O-toluidine) can cause methaemoglobinaemia. The maximum safe dose is:

- 6 mg/kg, maximum 400 mg (without adrenaline);
- 8 mg/kg, maximum 600 mg (with adrenaline).

Bupivacaine (Marcain)

This is a more recently introduced amide local anaesthetic agent, and is approximately four times as potent as lignocaine. It is used mainly for nerve blocks, epidural and spinal anaesthesia and is available as 0.25%, 0.5% and 0.75% solutions, the first two plus or minus adrenaline. Onset is relatively slow, and may take 30 minutes for a full effect when used epidurally, but it has a long duration of action, lasting up to 10 hours after a nerve block. It is widely used in obstetric analgesia, both epidurally and for spinals, as only low concentrations of drug cross the placenta. The maximum safe dose with or without adrenaline is:

- 2 mg/kg, maximum 150 mg in any 4 hours.

EMLA

This is a eutectic mixture of local anaesthetics, lignocaine and prilocaine in equal proportions (25 mg of each per gram). It is applied as a cream to the skin and produces surface analgesia in approximately 60 minutes. It is used to reduce the pain associated with venepuncture in children.

Ametop

This is a topical preparation of 4% amethocaine. It is used like EMLA to produce surface analgesia, but in a slightly shorter time.

Vasoconstrictors

These are added to local anaesthetics to reduce the rate of absorption, reduce toxicity and extend their duration of action. This is most effective during infiltration anaesthesia and nerve blocks, but less effective in epidurals or spinals. The two drugs used for their vasoconstrictor properties are adrenaline and felypressin. Some authorities recommend that solutions containing vasoconstrictors should never be used intrathecally.

> Local anaesthetics containing vasoconstrictors must never be used around extremities (e.g. fingers, toes, penis), as the vasoconstriction can cause fatal tissue ischaemia.

Adrenaline

Only very small concentrations are required to obtain intense vasoconstriction (α-adrenergic effect). The concentration present in solution is expressed as the weight of adrenaline (g) per volume of solution (ml). The concentrations commonly used range from $1 : 80\,000$ to $1 : 200\,000$.

$1 : 80\,000 = 1\,g$ in $80\,000\,ml = 1\,mg$ in $80\,ml = 0.0125\,mg/ml$ or $12.5\,\mu g/ml$.

$1 : 200\,000 = 1\,g$ in $200\,000\,ml = 1\,mg$ in $200\,ml = 0.005\,mg/ml$ or $5\,\mu g/ml$.

The maximum safe dose in an adult is $250\,\mu g$, i.e. 20 ml of $1 : 80\,000$ or 50 ml of $1 : 200\,000$. This should be reduced by 50% in patients with ischaemic heart disease.

Felypressin

This is a synthetic compound related to vasopressin (antidiuretic hormone (ADH)) with only vasoconstrictor properties. It is relatively safer for use in patients with heart disease. It is most commonly used in conjunction with prilocaine which contains 0.03 international units per ml (i.u./ml).

CALCULATION OF DOSES

For any drug it is essential that the correct dose is given and the maximum safe dose is never exceeded. This can be confusing with local anaesthetic drugs as the volume containing the required dose will vary depending upon the concentration which is expressed in per cent. Furthermore, a range of concentrations exist for each agent. The relationship between concentration, volume and dose is given by the formula:

$$\text{concentration}\,(\%) \times \text{volume}\,(ml) \times 10 = \text{dose}\,(mg).$$

THE CAUSES AND MANAGEMENT OF OVERDOSE

Overdose usually occurs for one of the following three reasons.

1 *Rapid absorption of a normally safe dose.* Use of an excessively concentrated solution or injection into a vascular area results in rapid absorption. It can also occur during IVRA if the tourniquet is released too soon or accidentally.

2 *Inadvertent i.v. injection.* Failure to aspirate prior to injection via virtually any route.

3 *Administration of a toxic dose.* Due to failure or error in calculating the maximum safe dose or failure to take into account any pre-existing cardiac or hepatic disease.

Signs and symptoms of overdose are due to effects on the central nervous system and the cardiovascular system. These are dependent on the plasma concentration and initially may represent either a mild overdose or more significantly, the early stages of a severe overdose.

• *Mild or early:* circumoral paraesthesia, numbness of the tongue, visual disturbances, lightheadedness, slurred speech, twitching, restlessness, mild hypotension and bradycardia.

• *Severe or late:* grand mal convulsions followed by coma, respiratory depression and eventually apnoea, cardiovascular collapse with profound hypotension and bradycardia, and ultimately cardiac arrest.

Management of overdose

If a patient complains of any the above symptoms or exhibits signs, then administration of local anaesthetic must cease immediately.

• *Airway.* Maintain using basic techniques. Tracheal intubation will be needed if the protective reflexes are absent, to protect against aspiration.

• *Breathing.* A high inspired concentration of oxygen (100%) is administered with support of ventilation if inadequate.

• *Circulation.* Raise the patient's legs to encourage venous return and start an i.v. infusion of crystalloid or colloid. Bradycardias should be treated with i.v. atropine. If no major pulse is palpable then commence external cardiac compression. If inotropes and vasopressors are required, invasive monitoring will be required and this should be performed on the intensive care unit.

• *Convulsions.* These must be treated early. Diazepam 5–10 mg intravenously can be used initially but this may cause significant respiratory depression. If the convulsions do not respond or they recur, then seek assistance.

Because of the risk of an inadvertent overdose of a local anaesthetic agent, they should only be administered where there are full facilities for resuscitation and monitoring immediately to hand. In this way the patient will recover without any permanent sequelae.

Local and regional anaesthetic techniques

Small, discrete areas of analgesia can be achieved either by topical application of a local anaesthetic agent, for example to the mucous membranes of the eye or urethra, or by subcutaneous infiltration (local analgesia). Larger areas of the body, such as a limb, can be anaesthetized by using local anaesthetic agents (regional anaesthesia) in several ways.

1 Intravenously after the application of a tourniquet (Bier's block).
2 Directly around nerves, for example the brachial plexus.
3 In the extradural space ('epidural anaesthesia').
4 In the subarachnoid space ('spinal anaesthesia').

The latter two techniques are more correctly called 'central neural blockade', however the term 'spinal anaesthesia' is commonly used when local anaesthetic is injected into the subarachnoid space and it is in this context that it will be used. The following is a brief introduction to some of the more popular regional anaesthetic techniques, those who require more detail should consult the texts in Further reading.

THE ROLE OF LOCAL AND REGIONAL ANAESTHESIA

Regional anaesthesia is not just a solution to the problem of anaesthesia in patients regarded as not well enough for general anaesthesia. The decision to use these techniques should be based on the advantages offered to both the patient and surgeon. The following are some of the considerations taken into account.

• Analgesia or anaesthesia is provided predominantly in the area required, thereby avoiding the systemic administration of drugs.

• In patients with chronic respiratory disease, spontaneous ventilation can be preserved and respiratory depressant drugs avoided.

• There is generally less disturbance of the control of coexisting systemic disease requiring medical therapy, for example diabetes mellitus.

• The airway reflexes are preserved and in a patient with a full stomach, particularly due to delayed gastric emptying (e.g. pregnancy), the risk of aspiration is reduced.

• Spinal and epidural anaesthesia may improve access and facilitate surgery, for example by causing contraction of the bowel or by providing profound muscle relaxation.

• Blood loss can be reduced with controlled hypotension.

• There is a considerable reduction in the equipment required and the cost of anaesthesia. This may be important in underdeveloped areas.

• When used in conjunction with general anaesthesia, only sufficient anaesthetic (inhalational or i.v.) is required to maintain unconsciousness, with analgesia and muscle relaxation provided by the regional technique.
• Some techniques can be continued postoperatively to provide pain relief, for example an epidural.

A patient should never be forced against their will to accept a local or regional technique. Initial objections and fears are best alleviated, and usually overcome, by explanation of the advantages and reassurance.

Whenever a local or regional anaesthetic technique is used, facilities for resuscitation must always be immediately available in order that allergic reactions and toxicity can be dealt with effectively. At a minimum this will include the following:
• Equipment to maintain and secure the airway, oxygen and a device for ventilation. Often this consists of an anaesthetic machine, tracheal tubes and breathing system.
• Intravenous cannulae and a range of fluids.
• Drugs, including adrenaline, atropine, vasopressors and anticonvulsants.
• Suction.
• The patient should be on a surface capable of being tipped head-down.

INFILTRATION ANALGESIA

A low concentration of local anaesthetic drug is injected subcutaneously, for example lignocaine 0.5%. If a large amount or a prolonged effect is required, then a solution containing adrenaline can be used, providing that tissues around end arteries are avoided. Infiltration analgesia is not instantaneous and lack of patience is the commonest reason for failure.

Method

1 Calculate the maximum volume of drug that can be used.
2 Clean the surrounding skin with an appropriate agent and allow to dry.
3 Insert the needle subcutaneously, avoiding any obvious blood vessels.
4 Aspirate to ensure that the tip of the needle does not lie in a blood vessel.
5 Inject the local anaesthetic in a constant flow as the needle is withdrawn. Too rapid injection will cause pain.
6 Second and subsequent punctures should be made through an area of skin already anaesthetized.

For removal of skin lesions, local anaesthetic is injected fanwise in the above manner from single punctures either side of the lesion (Fig. 8.1). For suturing, the needle is inserted into an area of intact skin at one

LOCAL INFILTRATION

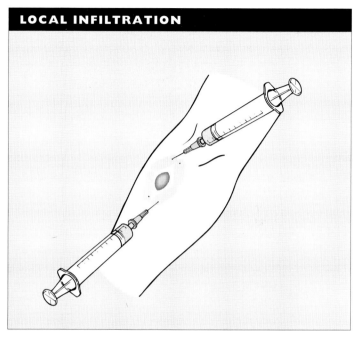

Fig. 8.1 Local infiltration.

end of the wound and advanced parallel to the wound, then local anaesthetic is injected as described. Alternatively, in a clean wound, local anaesthetic can be injected directly into the exposed wound edge. This technique can be used at the end of surgery to help reduce wound pain postoperatively.

INTRAVENOUS REGIONAL ANALGESIA (IVRA)

This technique is often referred to as a Bier's block after August Bier who first described it in 1908. Local anaesthetic is injected into the veins of an exsanguinated limb and retained by using an arterial tourniquet (Fig. 8.2). Preservative-free prilocaine without adrenaline is used, usually 30–40 ml of 0.5–1%. Anaesthesia is produced in 10–15 minutes and the duration is limited by discomfort caused by the tourniquet. Sensation returns soon after release of the tourniquet. This is a particularly useful technique for surgery of the distal upper limb.

Contraindications

These are relatively few but include patients with impaired peripheral circulation or sickle-cell disease.

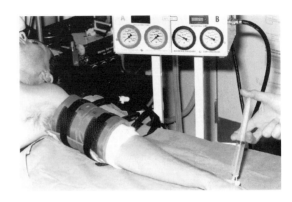

Fig. 8.2 Bier's block.

THE BRACHIAL PLEXUS

The nerves of the brachial plexus can be blocked with local anaesthetic agents above the level of the clavicle (supraclavicular brachial plexus block). With this approach, there is a risk of puncturing the apical pleura and causing a pneumothorax, and an alternative is the axillary approach. The median, ulnar and radial nerves enter the arm through the axilla within a fibrous sheath, along with the axillary artery and vein. The aim is to inject local anaesthetic drug within the sheath to block the nerves at this level. Often a nerve stimulator is attached to the needle to locate the nerves more precisely. Lignocaine, prilocaine or bupivacaine with adrenaline can be used. For a successful block, it is necessary to restrict distal spread and a tourniquet is applied (Fig. 8.3). This technique can be used for a wide range of surgical procedures below the elbow and will frequently provide good analgesia in the immediate postoperative period. As the block may last several hours, it is important to warn both the surgeon and patient of this.

EPIDURAL AND SPINAL ANAESTHESIA

These are probably the two most widely used regional anaesthetic techniques. Epidural (extradural) anaesthesia involves the deposition of a local anaesthetic drug into the potential space *outside* the dura. Spinal (intrathecal) anaesthesia results from the injection of a local anaesthetic drug directly into the cerebrospinal fluid (CSF), within the subarachnoid space. Until recently, epidural anaesthesia had the advantage that a catheter could be inserted allowing repeated injections to prolong the effect, whereas spinal anaesthesia was associated with a single injection and limited duration of action. A microcatheter is now available which can be placed in the subarachnoid space to allow repeated injections in a similar manner to epidurals.

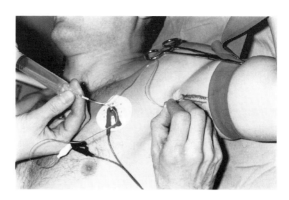

Fig. 8.3 Brachial plexus block via the axillary approach. The position of the artery is marked for clarity, and a nerve stimulator is being used.

The epidural space extends from the craniocervical junction at C1 to the sacrococcygeal membrane, and anaesthesia can theoretically be safely instituted at any level in between. In practice, it is most commonly performed in the lumbar region due to its ease and relative safety. Spinal anaesthesia is restricted to between the second lumbar and first sacral vertebrae, the upper limit is determined by the termination of the spinal cord, and the lower limit by the fact that the sacral vertebrae are fused and access becomes virtually impossible.

Epidural anaesthesia

Equipment and drugs

• The mainstay of the epidural is the Tuohy needle (16–18 gauge). This has a curved, blunt (Huber) point, with the terminal opening projecting sideways in an attempt to reduce the risk of dural puncture and facilitate the passage of a catheter into the epidural space (Fig. 8.4). The needle is marked at 3, 4, 5, 6 and 7 cm.

• To aid identification of the epidural space, a technique termed 'loss of resistance' is used. The Tuohy needle is advanced until its tip is embedded within the ligamentum flavum (yellow ligament). This causes marked resistance to attempted injection of either air or saline from a syringe attached to the needle. As the needle is advanced further, the ligament is pierced, resistance disappears dramatically and the air or saline is easily injected. To improve the sensitivity of this method, a syringe whose plunger moves with very low friction is manufactured (Fig. 8.4).

• The plastic catheter inserted into the epidural space via the Tuohy needle is marked at 5 cm intervals to 20 cm and at 1 cm intervals between 5 and 15 cm and has a terminal hole and several side holes within 2 cm of the tip (Fig. 8.4).

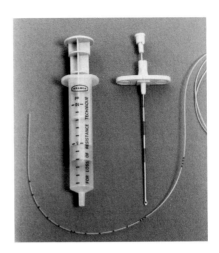

Fig. 8.4 Equipment for epidural: loss of resistance syringe; Tuohy needle and catheter.

- Bupivacaine 0.25–0.75% is widely used, weak solutions providing predominantly analgesia, and muscle relaxation increasing with concentration. The maximum safe dose remains at 2 mg/kg, thereby allowing 25–30 ml of 0.5% to be used in an average adult. Anaesthesia is generally established in 15–30 minutes and lasts 3–6 hours.

There is a small risk of the catheter inadvertently puncturing the dura as it is inserted down the Tuohy needle, and if a large volume of local anaesthetic drug is then injected, a proportion may end up in the CSF, resulting in very extensive spinal anaesthesia. To reduce this risk, a small volume (3–4 ml) of local anaesthetic is first injected, termed a 'test dose'. The patient is then observed for signs of a rapid-onset spinal-type anaesthetic which would result from the injection of this dose into the CSF.

Factors affecting the spread of an epidural anaesthetic

Local anaesthetic will spread from the level of injection both up and down the epidural space. The extent of anaesthesia is determined predominantly by the following:

- The spinal level of insertion of the epidural.
- The volume of local anaesthetic injected. Spread is greater in the thoracic region than in the lumbar region for a given volume. As most epidurals are performed in the lumbar region, a larger volume of local anaesthetic solution will be required for a higher level of anaesthesia and injected incrementally to achieve the appropriate level. For example:

    (a) 15–20 ml of 0.5% bupivacaine will provide anaesthesia to the T10 dermatome, sufficient for operations on the hip;

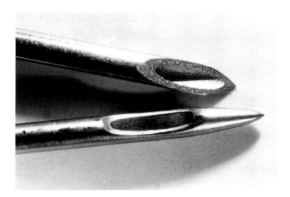

Fig. 8.5 Photomicrograph showing shape of bevel needle (top) and 'pencil point' needle (below). Courtesy of the *British Journal of Radiology*.

(b) 25–30 ml of 0.5% bupivacaine will provide anaesthesia to the T4 dermatome for abdominal operations.
• Gravity: tipping the patient head-down encourages spread cranially, head-up tends to limit spread.

The spread of anaesthesia is described with reference to the limits of the dermatomes affected. In practice, often only the upper limit is determined, for example: the inguinal ligament, T12; the umbilicus, T10; and the nipples, T4.

Spinal anaesthesia

Equipment and drugs
• A fine, 22–29 gauge needle with either a traditional bevel (Quincke) point or a tapered, 'pencil point' (Whitacre, Sprotte) is used (Fig. 8.5). The small diameter and shape are an attempt to reduce the incidence of post-dural puncture headache (see below).
• To aid passage of the needle through the skin and interspinous ligament, a short, wide-bore needle is introduced initially and the spinal needle passed through its lumen.
• Hyperbaric bupivacaine 0.5% is widely used (i.e. its specific gravity is greater than CSF), this is achieved by the addition of 8% dextrose. It is often referred to as 'heavy bupivacaine'. Adrenaline-containing solutions are not used because of the risk of vasoconstriction compromising the spinal cord blood flow.

Factors affecting the spread of a spinal anaesthetic
Many factors influence the spread of the local anaesthetic drug within the CSF and hence the extent of anaesthesia.

- Increasing the dose (volume or concentration) of local anaesthetic drug rapidly saturates the nerves.
- The higher the spinal anaesthetic is performed in the lumbar region, the higher the level of block obtained.
- Positioning of the patient after injection is used to influence the extent of anaesthesia. Maintenance of the sitting position after injection results in a block of the low lumbar and sacral nerves. In the supine position, the block will extend to the thoracic nerves to around T5–6, the point of maximum backwards curve (kyphosis) of the thoracic spine. Further extension can be obtained with a head-down tilt.

Monitoring during local and regional anaesthesia

The fact that the patient remains conscious is not a reason for inadequate monitoring. During epidural and spinal anaesthesia, particular attention should be paid to the cardiovascular system as a result of the profound effects these techniques can have. Maintenance of verbal contact with the patient is useful as it gives an indication of cerebral perfusion. Early signs of an inadequate cardiac output are often the patient complaining of nausea, faintness and subsequently vomiting. The first indication of extensive spread of anaesthesia may be a complaint of difficulty with breathing or numbness in the fingers. Clearly, these valuable signs and symptoms will be lost if the patient is heavily sedated.

Complications of central neural blockade

Although there is a large list of complications associated with these techniques, they are frequently mild and rarely cause any lasting morbidity. The incidence of the ones most common with spinal anaesthesia is shown in Table 8.1.

Hypotension and bradycardia

These occur secondary to sympathetic block. Loss of sympathetic tone reduces the peripheral resistance, and venodilatation reduces venous return to the heart. If the block extends cranially beyond T5, the sympathetic nerves to the heart responsible for increasing heart rate are blocked, leaving the vagal tone unopposed and resulting in a bradycardia. If the blood pressure falls (>30% resting value) it is usually treated by administering oxygen via a facemask, and i.v. fluids (crystalloids or colloids) to increase venous return. Vasopressors, commonly ephedrine (α- and β-agonist) may be used to counteract the peripheral vasodilatation. A bradycardia will usually respond to 0.3–0.6 mg atropine given intravenously.

Nausea and vomiting

These mostly occur as a result of hypotension and cerebral hypoxia, but

INCIDENCE OF COMMON COMPLICATIONS	
Hypotension	33%
Nausea	18%
Bradycardia	13%
Vomiting	7%
Dysrhythmias	2%

Table 8.1 Incidence of common complications during spinal anaesthesia.

can also result from vagal stimulation during upper abdominal surgery. Any hypotension or hypoxia is corrected as described above. If due to surgery, try to reduce the degree of manipulation. If this is not possible then it may be necessary to convert to general anaesthesia. Atropine 0.3–0.6 mg is frequently effective, particularly if there is a bradycardia. Anti-emetics can be tried (e.g. metoclopramide 10 mg intravenously), but this must not be at the expense of the above.

Postdural puncture headache

This is thought to be due primarily to a persistent leakage of CSF from a hole made in the lumbar dura. The incidence is greatest with large holes, i.e. when a hole is made accidentally with a Tuohy needle. The incidence after spinal anaesthesia can be minimized by using very fine needles (e.g. 26 gauge) or ones with a 'pencil point'. The patient usually complains of a headache which is frontal or occipital, postural, worse when standing and exacerbated by straining. The majority of headaches will resolve spontaneously.

Contraindications to epidural and spinal anaesthesia

- Hypovolaemia either as a result of blood loss or dehydration. Such patients are likely to experience severe falls in blood pressure as compensatory vasoconstriction is lost.
- A low, fixed cardiac output as seen with severe aortic or mitral stenosis. The reduced venous return further reduces cardiac output, jeopardizing perfusion of vital organs.
- Local skin sepsis because of the risk of introducing infection.
- Where coagulation is abnormal, either as a result of a bleeding diathesis (e.g. haemophilia) or therapeutic anticoagulation, there is the risk of causing an epidural haematoma. There may also be a very small risk in patients taking aspirin and associated drugs which reduce platelet activity. Where heparin is used perioperatively to reduce the risk of deep venous thrombosis, then this may be started after the insertion of the epidural or spinal.

- Raised intracranial pressure because of the risk of precipitating coning.
- Known allergy to amide local anaesthetic drugs.
- A patient who is totally uncooperative.
- Where there is concurrent disease of the CNS, some would caution against the use of these techniques for fear of being blamed for any subsequent deterioration.
- Although not an absolute contraindication, the performance of epidural or spinal anaesthesia may be technically difficult in those patients who have had previous spinal surgery or have abnormal spinal anatomy.

Further reading

Carpenter RL, Caplan RA, Brown DL *et al.* Incidence and risk factors for side effects of spinal anesthesia. *Anesthesiology* 1992; **76**: 906–19.

Hickey R, Ramamurthy S. Brachial plexus block. *Current Opinion in Anaesthesiology* 1993; **6** (5): 823–9.

Lee JA, Atkinson RS, Watt MJ. *Sir Robert Macintosh's Lumbar Puncture and Spinal Analgesia*, 5th edn. Edinburgh: Churchill Livingstone, 1985.

Wildsmith JAW, Armitage EN (eds). *Principles and Practice of Regional Anaesthesia*. Edinburgh: Churchill Livingstone, 1990.

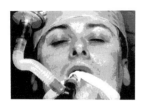

Putting it All Together

The information presented so far has divided anaesthesia into distinct stages, looking at how each may be achieved individually. In clinical practice, no such clear divide exists; anaesthesia is a continuum from induction to recovery. Irrespective of the technique used, successful general anaesthesia has three characteristic components which must be achieved.

1 *Narcosis:* the term used to describe that the patient is unconscious, unaware of the surgical procedure and has no recall on regaining consciousness.

2 *Reflex suppression:* both somatic and autonomic. As a result of the former, the patient does not respond to surgery (as one normally would to a painful stimulus) and the potentially harmful sympathetic responses, for example tachycardia and hypertension are suppressed.

3 *Muscle relaxation:* of varying degrees to facilitate surgical access.

It is important to look at how these key features are achieved using the two main general anaesthetic techniques for elective surgery and finally the main differences for emergency surgery. The following is intended as an overview, not a detailed account of the conduct of a general anaesthetic!

Anaesthesia for elective surgery

SPONTANEOUS VENTILATION

On arrival in the anaesthetic room, simple monitoring will take place (electrocardiogram (ECG), blood pressure, pulse oximetry) and venous access is established. The patient is then preoxygenated by breathing 100% oxygen via the anaesthetic system and an intravenous (i.v.) induction agent is administered. Once consciousness is lost, the inspired mixture is changed to one containing oxygen, nitrous oxide and a volatile anaesthetic agent in order to maintain anaesthesia. A short period of apnoea is not uncommon and if prolonged (> 45–60 seconds), manual ventilation is performed until spontaneous ventilation is resumed. Gradually, the inspired concentration of the volatile agent is increased, taking care not to induce coughing, until anaesthesia is deep enough to allow surgery (i.e. somatic reflex suppression occurs). The airway is maintained manually using a jaw thrust, frequently supplemented with an oropharyngeal or nasopharyngeal airway. Alternatively, a laryngeal mask may be used.

The patient is then transferred to the operating theatre and monitoring continued as in the anaesthetic room, with the possible addition of monitoring the inspired concentration of oxygen and anaesthetic agent. After positioning the patient appropriately, surgery commences and the concentration of the volatile agent is adjusted according to the patient's response to surgery.

This technique of general anaesthesia is reserved mainly for peripheral surgery where significant muscle relaxation is not required and autonomic reflexes can be modified by the careful titration of i.v. opioid analgesics.

Towards the end of surgery, the concentration of volatile agent is gradually reduced as the surgical stimulus allows. Nitrous oxide is eventually discontinued and the patient breathes 100% oxygen. An increased inspired oxygen concentration is continued into the recovery area to counter the diffusion hypoxia caused by the excretion of nitrous oxide and to compensate for any hypoventilation. The patient is turned onto their side and as the laryngeal reflexes return, any airway adjunct removed.

An alternative to this technique is the use of a total i.v. anaesthesia, where an i.v. agent is substituted for the volatile agent while the patient breathes either oxygen-enriched air or oxygen and nitrous oxide.

A local or regional anaesthetic technique is frequently used to supplement general anaesthesia in a spontaneously breathing patient. This will provide analgesia and muscle relaxation and allow the use of a lower concentration of volatile agent or a reduced rate of infusion of an i.v. agent.

CONTROLLED VENTILATION

The initial steps of monitoring, preoxygenation and venous access are as already described. Following i.v. induction, it is good practice to ensure that the patient's lungs can be manually ventilated as the next stage is the use of a muscle relaxant to facilitate intubation of the trachea. Should this prove unexpectedly difficult or impossible, then at least the operator knows that oxygenation can be maintained. After the relaxant has been given, an i.v. opioid analgesic is often administered.

During the period it takes for the (non-depolarizing) muscle relaxant to achieve its desired effect, the patient is manually ventilated with the anaesthetic system delivering oxygen, nitrous oxide and a volatile agent to ensure oxygenation and maintenance of anaesthesia. Once neuromuscular block is considered adequate, laryngoscopy is performed and the trachea intubated. Again the patient is usually manually ventilated at this stage while the position of the tube is checked by watching chest movement, auscultation of breath sounds and possibly measuring the carbon dioxide concentration in expired gas. Finally, the tube is secured with adhesive tape or bandage. If further anaesthetic procedures are required, for example insertion of a central venous pressure (CVP) catheter, then the patient is connected to a mechanical ventilator in the anaesthetic room, otherwise the patient is transferred to the operating theatre.

Once in the theatre, the first manoeuvre must be to connect the patient to the ventilator and check to ensure that the tracheal tube has not become displaced and that the lungs are being adequately ventilated. Monitoring is commenced as described above, but in addition a ventilator disconnect alarm is included and the intensity of neuromuscular block is monitored. Finally, the patient is positioned and surgery allowed to start.

Using this technique, specific drugs are used to achieve each of the three components of general anaesthesia: (i) low concentration of a volatile agent (or alternatively a constant infusion of an i.v. agent) is used to ensure unconsciousness; (ii) autonomic reflexes are modified by the use of a potent analgesic; and (iii) the use of a muscle relaxant prevents somatic reflexes and provides profound relaxation to facilitate surgical access. Each component is therefore achieved independently and tailored towards the needs of the patient, surgeon and anaesthetist. This minimizes any unwanted side-effects, particularly those attributable to the excess administration of the volatile agent. This technique of anaesthesia is often referred to as 'balanced anaesthesia'.

During surgery, incremental doses of relaxants and analgesics can be given according to the patient's response. As described in the previous section, a regional anaesthetic technique is sometimes used to provide the analgesic component.

At the end of surgery, any residual neuromuscular block is reversed, the volatile agent (or i.v. infusion) and nitrous oxide is discontinued and the patient ventilated with 100% oxygen. The pharynx is suctioned to remove any secretions and on return of spontaneous ventilation and the laryngeal reflexes, the patient is extubated, preferably on their side.

POSITIONING THE PATIENT

Prior to surgery, the patient is placed in a position to facilitate access. Sufficient theatre staff must be assembled to carry out this task safely and any additional equipment required must be assembled and to hand before any manoeuvring of the patient begins. The overall positioning of the patient is carried out under the direction (and with the assistance) of the anaesthetist, with the prime concern being the safety of the patient. Detailed adjustment is usually carried out in conjunction with the surgeon. Finally, before covering the patient with the surgical drapes, the adequacy of ventilation, monitoring and intravascular access must be checked. The three most common positions used are: supine; lateral; and prone.

• When supine, the patient lies flat on their back, with their head and neck in a neutral position. The arms are placed either along the patient's sides or flexed at the elbows to lie across the lower chest. Occasionally, one arm is placed at the side while the other is abducted (<90°) and supported on an arm board. The legs are extended in a neutral position. In gynaecological and urological surgery, the hips and knees are flexed to 90°, legs abducted slightly and the ankles supported in stirrups.

• The lateral position is relatively unstable, requiring a variety of supports to ensure the safety of the patient and which are placed according to the site of surgery. During mechanical ventilation, the upper lung is preferentially ventilated, while the dependent lung receives a greater blood flow. This can result in a marked reduction in oxygenation which is exacerbated by pre-existing pulmonary disease and therefore a greater degree of monitoring is often used for patients in this position.

• Many variations have evolved of the prone position using specially designed frames, props and supports which generally support the chest and pelvis leaving the abdomen free. One problem is profound hypotension secondary to badly placed supports reducing venous return and the cardiac output. Close monitoring of the cardiovascular system is essential both during turning and intraoperatively.

Anaesthesia for emergency surgery

When faced with a patient requiring emergency surgery the anaesthetic technique is modified slightly as it is assumed that the patient will have a 'full stomach' and there is an increased risk of regurgitation, and in the absence of the laryngeal reflexes, aspiration into the lungs. Consequently, the majority of patients will be intubated in order to protect their airway.

RAPID-SEQUENCE INDUCTION OF ANAESTHESIA

Preoxygenation commences using high-flow oxygen delivered via the anaesthetic system and the patient is encouraged to apply the mask with a good fit to their face. This should be maintained for 3 minutes, during which time monitors are applied and venous access established, and an i.v.

infusion is started. The suction apparatus is switched on and a rigid Yankeur sucker attached and placed within immediate reach of the anaesthetist. A check is made that the anaesthetic assistant is able to apply cricoid pressure effectively and that they understand it is not to be released until instruction is given by the anaesthetist (see Fig. 3.8). Finally, the patient is warned about the feeling of pressure on their neck as they loose consciousness.

The i.v. induction agent is administered and as consciousness is lost, cricoid pressure is applied and the suxamethonium is administered. The facemask is held against the patient's face but manual ventilation is not performed to avoid the risk of distending the stomach and increasing the risk of regurgitation. Once the fasciculations have stopped, laryngoscopy is performed and the patient intubated. The cuff is inflated and the position of the tracheal tube is checked as already described. Only when the anaesthetist is confident that the tube is in the trachea is the cricoid pressure released.

The only deviation from this plan is if the patient begins to actively vomit, in which case instruction must be given to release the cricoid pressure in order to reduce the risk of oesophageal rupture as a result of the high pressures which can be generated. The patient should then be turned laterally if it is safe to do so, and the pharynx aspirated.

The anaesthetic and surgery then continue as described previously for elective surgery. A non-depolarizing relaxant is administered either when there is clinical evidence that the effects of the suxamethonium are wearing off or as indicated by monitoring neuromuscular blockade with a peripheral nerve stimulator. It is not unusual to pass a nasogastric (or orogastric) tube during surgery to reduce the volume of the gastric contents. However, this does not guarantee that the stomach is empty. Therefore, at the end of surgery, whenever possible, it is always safer to extubate the patient on their side and leave them in this position until they have fully regained consciousness and their laryngeal reflexes.

Further reading

Anderton JM, Keen RI, Neave R. *Positioning the Surgical Patient.* London: Butterworths, 1988.

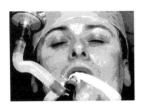

An Introduction to Intensive Care

The intensive care unit (ICU) is a designated area within a hospital where specialized treatment of critically ill patients takes place. In order to achieve this, there is a concentration of resources including: a wide range of complex monitoring equipment, mechanical ventilators, facilities for organ support, and the use of potent drugs which are often given by continuous intravenous (i.v.) infusion. Complementing or in lieu of the ICU, there may be a high dependency unit (HDU) where the level of care is intermediate between that found on the ICU and the general ward. Patients suffering from acute myocardial infarction are generally admitted to specialized coronary care units (CCU) while neurosurgical and head-injured patients may be admitted to a specialized area of the neurosurgical ward for short periods of mechanical ventilation.

It is recommended that 1–2% of the total number of acute hospital beds should be located in the ICU. The ideal size for an ICU is four to ten beds and smaller units may be inefficient in their use of resources. It has been suggested that in order to maximize clinical and financial efficiency, much larger regional ICUs should be established. The challenge for those involved in the care of critically ill patients is to aim resources at those patients likely to survive, by providing artificial support of one or more failing physiological systems until natural recuperation and/or therapeutically assisted recovery can take place. Patients may be admitted to the ICU electively following major surgery, or as medical or surgical emergencies. In an attempt to differentiate potential survivors from non-survivors, a number of 'scoring systems' have been developed which take account of various aspects of the patient's acute physiological upset, their age and any chronic health problems (e.g. APACHE II). However, they are not yet sufficiently accurate to be used as the sole basis for deciding whether or not to treat an *individual* patient.

Monitoring on the intensive care unit

Physiological monitoring is an essential aid in the diagnosis and management of critically ill patients, in evaluating their response to treatment and alerting staff to the onset of a sudden deterioration in the patient's condition. There is a spectrum of monitoring. At its most basic level it comprises clinical observation and examination (for which there is still no substitute), extending to complex, invasive methods for the measurement of haemodynamic and oxygen transport variables, etc.

ELECTROCARDIOGRAM

All patients should have a continuously displayed electrocardiogram (ECG) for the detection of acute dysrhythmias, and to a lesser extent (except on the CCU) acute ischaemia (Table 9.1). In critically ill patients, supraventricular tachycardias predominate, especially atrial fibrillation.

ARTERIAL BLOOD PRESSURE

Systemic arterial blood pressure is normally closely regulated in order to maintain an adequate pressure to ensure tissue perfusion. Although the

AETIOLOGY OF CARDIAC DYSRHYTHMIAS

Electrolyte disturbances
  Hypokalaemia
  Hyperkalaemia
  Hypocalcaemia
  Hypomagnesaemia
  Acid–base disturbances
Drugs
  Inotropes
  Bronchodilators
  Antidysrhythmics
  β-blockers, Ca-antagonists
  Diuretics
  Overdosage of antidepressants
Pre-existing ischaemic heart disease
Hypoxia
Cardiotoxic effects of sepsis

Table 9.1 Aetiology of cardiac dysrhythmias in critically ill patients.

normal values tend to increase with age, mean arterial pressure (MAP) should be maintained above a minimum value of 60 mmHg. MAP is dependent on cardiac output and systemic vascular resistance (SVR). Measurement of arterial blood pressure is thus a relatively crude *indicator* of cardiac performance and circulatory flow, as it may be normal or elevated in the presence of a low cardiac output and poor tissue perfusion. Interpretation of the blood pressure must be taken in the context of other clinical measurements and in critically ill patients it is more useful to measure the cardiac output itself (see below).

Arterial blood pressure is usually monitored directly in the ICU as it is more accurate, it is continuous and the presence of an indwelling cannula in an artery allows blood sampling without the need for repeated puncturing of veins or arteries. The advantages and disadvantages of direct measurement are shown in Table 9.2.

A cannula is inserted percutaneously into a suitable artery, frequently the radial artery of the non-dominant hand (alternatives being the femoral, dorsalis pedis, brachial and axillary arteries). The arterial blood pressure is transmitted via a saline-filled catheter to a pressure transducer which converts the mechanical signal to a very small electrical signal, proportional to the pressure. This signal is amplified and displayed on a monitor as both a waveform and pressure readings, systolic, diastolic and mean. In order to ensure the readings are accurate, the system is zeroed by exposing the transducer to atmosphere and ensuring that the monitor

ADVANTAGES AND DISADVANTAGES

Advantages	Disadvantages
Accuracy	Complex to perform
Continuous measurement gives immediate warning of important changes in blood pressure	Potentially inaccurate if apparatus is not set up correctly
	Haematoma at puncture site
Shape of arterial waveform gives information relating to myocardial contractility and other haemodynamic variables	Infection at puncture site/ bacteraemia/septicaemia
	Disconnection haemorrhage
Facility for frequent arterial blood sampling	Embolization
	Arterial thrombosis

Table 9.2 Advantages and disadvantages of direct arterial blood pressure measurement.

reads zero pressure. To prevent the system becoming blocked, it is flushed constantly with heparinized saline at 3 ml/hour from a pressurized source to prevent backflow. Central venous and pulmonary artery pressures are measured using the same system.

CENTRAL VENOUS PRESSURE

The central venous pressure (CVP) is an index of the patient's circulating volume (or more correctly right ventricular preload). It is useful for directing fluid therapy in cases of dehydration, hypovolaemia due to haemorrhage and sepsis syndrome, and in the diagnosis and management of heart failure. The routes commonly used to measure the CVP are discussed on page 97. A central venous cannula is used for a variety of other purposes in the ITU as shown in Table 9.3.

The main limitation in monitoring CVP is that, by definition, therapy is directed towards optimizing the filling pressures on the right side of the heart. While the filling pressures of the right and left sides are normally closely related, this relationship may not hold in critically ill patients, particularly those with pre-existing cardiac or respiratory disease. In this situation it is of greater therapeutic value to monitor and optimize conditions for the left ventricle.

PULMONARY ARTERY PRESSURES

Pressures in the pulmonary artery are monitored using a pulmonary artery flotation catheter (PAFC), sometimes referred to as a 'Swan–Ganz' catheter after its inventors. This is a multi-lumen catheter with an inflatable balloon and a temperature thermistor at its distal end.

A PAFC is inserted percutaneously via either the internal jugular or

---

USES OF CENTRAL VEIN CATHETERIZATION

Measurement of central venous pressure
Infusion of irritant solutions, e.g. KCl
Infusion of vasoconstrictor agents, e.g. noradrenaline, dopamine
Total parenteral nutrition
Route for insertion of temporary cardiac pacing wire
Route for insertion of pulmonary artery flotation catheter
Venous access for haemodialysis, haemofiltration, plasmaphoresis, etc.
Venous access in absence of peripheral veins
Venous access during cardiac arrest

Table 9.3 Uses of central vein catheterization.

subclavian veins in the same manner as inserting a CVP. It is advanced through the right atrium and ventricle until the tip lies in a main branch of the pulmonary artery. In this position, an indirect assessment of the filling pressure in the left ventricle can be made (referred to as the 'left ventricular end-diastolic pressure', LVEDP or preload), which is a more accurate indication of the patient's circulating volume than the CVP. The pressure is influenced by many of the factors affecting CVP and trends are more useful than absolute values. Complications associated with PAFC insertion are listed in Table 9.4.

In addition to this information, the catheter can also be used to measure cardiac output and allow mixed venous blood to be sampled. Recently, PAFCs have become available incorporating two fibreoptic channels to allow continuous measurement of mixed venous oxygen saturation. One channel transmits near infrared light which is reflected by the passing red cells; a second fibreoptic channel conducts the reflected light to a photodetector that determines the oxygen saturation of the haemoglobin.

PULSE OXIMETRY

The pulse oximeter provides a quick, non-invasive assessment of the oxygenation of the peripheral tissues (SpO_2). It therefore gives a simultaneous indication of the degree of oxygenation of the blood by the respiratory system and the ability of the cardiovascular system to deliver it to the tissues. By providing continuous monitoring it can be used to give an early warning of deterioration in the patient's condition. The principles of operation are described on page 84.

COMPLICATIONS

All of the complications associated with central venous catheterization
Ventricular dysrhythmias
Pulmonary infarction
Pulmonary artery rupture
Knot formation
Balloon rupture
Subacute bacterial endocarditis
Pericardial tamponade
Damage to tricuspid or pulmonary valve

Table 9.4 Complications of pulmonary artery catheterization.

TRANSOESOPHAGEAL ECHOCARDIOGRAPHY

Transoesophageal echocardiography (TOE) provides quite sophisticated information relating to ventricular and valvular function of the heart and cardiac output. The technique is relatively non-invasive: the apparatus consisting of a modified gastroscope placed in the oesophagus, behind the heart. Monitoring is continuous, and acute changes in cardiac performance or cardiac output can be detected. The role of TOE on the ICU is currently being evaluated.

RENAL FUNCTION

In critically ill patients, acute renal failure is a common problem due usually to either failure to maintain adequate renal perfusion (pre-renal) or intrinsic renal failure. Often the two are closely interlinked in aetiology (Table 9.5), but distinction may be helped by biochemical investigations (Table 9.6).

All patients on an ICU should have their plasma urea, creatinine and

AETIOLOGY OF ACUTE RENAL FAILURE

Pre-renal
Dehydration, e.g. vomiting, diarrhoea
Haemorrhage
Cardiogenic shock
'Third space losses' e.g. trauma, major surgery, bowel obstruction, etc.

Renal
Acute tubular necrosis (usually secondary to severe pre-renal failure)
Sepsis
Severe obstructive jaundice
Blood transfusion reaction
Myoglobinaemia
Peritonitis
'Medical' causes:
    Acute pyelonephritis
    Acute glomerulonephritis
    Acute pancreatitis
    Nephrotic syndrome
    Bowel obstruction
    Vasculitis
    Burns
    Renal vein thrombosis

Table 9.5 Aetiology of acute renal failure.

DIFFERENTIATION OF ACUTE RENAL FAILURE

Index	Pre-renal	Intrinsic renal
Urine concentration	High: specific gravity ≥ 1020; osmolarity > 550 mosmol/l	Dilute: specific gravity 1010; osmolarity < 350 mosmol/l
Urine [Na]	< 20 mmol/l	> 40 mmol/l
Urine/plasma osmolar ratio	$\geq 2:1$	$1.1:1$
Urine/plasma urea	$\geq 20:1$	$< 10:1$
Urine/plasma creatinine	$\geq 40:1$	$< 10:1$

Table 9.6 Differentiation of pre-renal from intrinsic renal failure.

electrolytes (Na, K, Ca, phosphate) measured at least once daily and urine output monitored hourly. Estimation of glomerular filtration rate (GFR) from the creatinine clearance (CL_{CR}) is a more precise index of renal function:

$$GFR \approx CR_{CL} = \frac{\text{rate of urinary output} \times \text{urine} \left[Cr \right]}{\text{plasma} \left[Cr \right]}.$$

NEUROLOGICAL ASSESSMENT

Neurological assessment of patients on the ICU is often difficult because of the use of sedatives and neuromuscular blocking drugs. Ideally, a minimal level of sedation should be employed, titrated for each individual and compatible with a comfortable, settled patient. The Glasgow coma scale can be used, provided that allowances are made for the effects of drugs and the presence of an endotracheal tube. Patients who have undergone major intracranial surgery or sustained a severe head injury may have their intracranial pressure (ICP) monitored using either an intraventricular catheter, or sensor placed in the subarachnoid extradural space. These are connected via a transducer to produce both a waveform and reading of the ICP. The aim is to keep the ICP below 20 mmHg whilst maintaining cerebral perfusion pressure (MAP — ICP) between 60 and 80 mmHg.

HEPATIC FUNCTION

Hepatic dysfunction may be primary, or more commonly in the context of intensive care, secondary to another disease process (Table 9.7). Liver

CAUSES OF HEPATIC DYSFUNCTION

Primary	Secondary
Viral hepatitis: A, B, C, CMV, EBV, etc.	Sepsis syndrome
Alcoholic liver disease	Hypoxia
Drug-induced hepatitis: halothane, sodium valproate, isoniazid, paracetamol overdosage	Hypotension
Autoimmune hepatitis/cirrhosis	Cardiac failure
Acute fatty liver of pregnancy	Cholestasis
Inborn error of metabolism, e.g. Wilson's disease	Cholangitis
CMV, cytomegalovirus; EBV, Epstein–Barr virus.	

Table 9.7 Causes of hepatic dysfunction.

function is monitored by serum bilirubin (conjugated/unconjugated), albumin, transaminases (AST, ALT, GGT), alkaline phosphatase, prothrombin time (PT) and activated partial thromboplastin time (APTT). The PT is probably the most sensitive indicator of hepatic reserve and prognosis in fulminant liver failure.

MISCELLANEOUS

Routine haematology (haemoglobin concentration, white cell count, platelet count) should be assessed daily. Trace elements (Cu, Mg, Zn, Se) may need monitoring in patients who are resident on the ICU for more than 1 week, particularly during parenteral nutrition. Serum lactate levels are measured on some ICUs as a more specific indicator of metabolic acidosis associated with tissue hypoxia, although the clinical advantages are disputed.

Mechanical ventilation on the intensive care unit

One of the commonest interventions on the ICU is mechanical ventilation of critically ill patients who have developed respiratory failure, or when it is thought imminent in an exhausted patient. Hypoxaemia (Pa_{O_2} <60 mmHg) with or without accompanying hypercapnia (Pa_{CO_2} >50 mmHg) is usually present despite high-flow oxygen via a facemask. The aim of mechanical ventilation is to optimize oxygenation of the patient and to allow a period of respite. The causes of respiratory failure are diverse (Table 9.8). A common presentation in patients admitted to the ICU is the so-called adult respiratory distress syndrome (ARDS). Following a variety of insults, the pulmonary capillaries become hyperpermeable, with leakage of fluid and the development of non-cardiogenic pulmonary oedema. This results in areas of ventilation/perfusion mismatch, severe hypoxaemia and physical exhaustion as the patient tries to compensate.

During mechanical ventilation, the distribution of gas flow through the lungs, the shape of the chest wall and the pattern and extent of diaphragmatic movement is altered. This tends to lead to a small increase in ventilation/perfusion mismatching. However, the net result of mechanical ventilation in patients with respiratory failure is usually beneficial in improving arterial Pao_2 and $Paco_2$ values (Table 9.9), and may also relieve a failing left ventricle and reduce cardiogenic pulmonary oedema. This is a result of a reduction in venous return to the heart reducing the preload, and in addition, a reduced afterload from the increased pressure gradient between the thoracic and abdominal aorta occurring during inspiration.

Critically ill patients requiring ventilation often have a reduction in lung compliance and an increase in resistance to respiratory gas flow. Consequently, ICU ventilators are principally electronically controlled and programmed to ensure that the desired tidal volume is delivered. To achieve this they have a much greater control of inspiratory gas flow and adjustment in the time taken for inspiration and expiration, usually expressed as the inspiratory:expiratory (I:E) ratio. Furthermore, a variety of modes are available which allow partial ventilation, usually synchronized with the patient's own efforts.

INTUBATION AND TRACHEOSTOMY

The majority of patients on the ICU are ventilated through a cuffed endotracheal tube inserted via the mouth or nose. The cuff should have a large volume to minimize the pressure exerted on the tracheal mucosa. Prolonged intubation can be uncomfortable and associated with difficult oral hygiene, infection and ulceration. If the period of ventilation extends beyond 7–10 days, it is usual to perform a tracheostomy. Until recently, a tracheostomy necessitated a formal procedure in the operating theatre, however, many tracheostomies are now created on the ICU using a percutaneous technique. In one such method, a series of progressively larger dilators are passed through a small incision in the trachea along a guidewire, until the track is large enough to accommodate the tracheostomy tube.

CAUSES OF RESPIRATORY FAILURE

Hypoventilation
Physical exhaustion
Diaphragmatic splinting due to acute abdominal or chest pain (often postsurgical)
CNS depression
    Drugs, e.g. opioids, sedatives
    Head injury
    Cerebral haemorrhage/tumour
Neuromuscular
    Myopathies
    Guillain–Barré syndrome
    Myasthenia gravis
Acute airway obstruction
    Laryngeal tumour
    Asthma
    Acute exacerbation COAD

Ventilation/perfusion imbalance
ARDS
Pulmonary consolidation
Pneumothorax/haemothorax
Disordered hypoxic-pulmonary vasoconstriction reflex
    Secondary to sepsis, vasoactive drugs
Collapse of small airways as FRC falls below closing lung volume
    Exhaustion
    Obesity
    Abdominal distension
    Abdominal pain
    Chest wall injury/pain
    Aspiration
    Viscid secretions
Pulmonary contusion
Cardiogenic pulmonary oedema
Pulmonary embolism

Diffusion defect at the alveolar-capillary membrane
Pulmonary fibrosis
Extrinsic allergic alveolitis
Emphysema

ARDS, adult respiratory distress syndrome; CNS, central nervous system; COAD, chronic obstructive airways disease; FRC, functional residual capacity.

Table 9.8 Causes of respiratory failure.

ADVANTAGES OF IPPV	
Problem in acute respiratory failure	**Result of IPPV**
Exhaustion of patient	Patient is sedated and the work of breathing is relieved
Poor toleration of face mask	
Difficult to supply >60% oxygen	Increase in inspired oxygen concentration up to 100%
Ventilation/perfusion mismatch increases as FRC reduced below the lung volume at which small airways collapse. Usually a result of exhaustion or diaphragmatic splinting due to pain or abdominal distension	Rapid, shallow breaths replaced by larger tidal volumes
	Application of a PEEP increases FRC
FRC, functional residual capacity; PEEP, positive end-expiratory pressure.	

Table 9.9 Advantages of IPPV in acute respiratory failure.

Sedation and analgesia

Critically ill patients admitted to the ICU require varying degrees of sedation and analgesia. These are not synonymous terms and require different drugs and techniques. Many critically ill patients are confused and disorientated by their illness and are likely to become agitated by their environment. For patients with insight, the realization of the seriousness of their condition and the contemplation of their own mortality can be frightening, and the psychological trauma engendered may actually hinder recovery. An appropriate level of sedation produces calm, co-operative patients who are thus easier to nurse and treat. Similarly, patients admitted to the ICU following major surgery or trauma will suffer if good analgesia is not provided. Some of the invasive procedures which are undertaken on patients are also painful and the presence of the endotracheal tube itself can be distressingly uncomfortable. As recently as 10–15 years ago, it was common practice to deeply sedate and paralyse patients so that they were completely unaware of their surroundings. It is now realized that such deep sedation is not only unnecessary, but may also be harmful (Table 9.10).

The ideal level of sedation is one in which the patient is calm, awake and orientated during appropriate periods of the day. The Ramsay sedation scale (Table 9.11) is used on many ICUs, a score of 2–4 being satisfactory depending on the clinical situation, time of day, etc.

PROBLEMS ASSOCIATED WITH DEEP SEDATION WITH PARALYSIS

Immunosuppression
Increased incidence of infection
Risk of awareness if sedation is inadequate
Prolonged recovery times
Loss of contact with reality, with an adverse effect on psychological well-being

Table 9.10 Problems associated with deep sedation with paralysis.

RAMSAY SEDATION SCALE

Level	Conscious level
1	Restless and agitated
2	Co-operative, calm, orientated
3	Asleep, responds to verbal command
4	Asleep, responds briskly to glabellar tap
5	Asleep, responds sluggishly to glabellar tap
6	No response

Table 9.11 Ramsay sedation scale.

The most commonly used sedative drugs are midazolam and propofol, although other drugs are used in specific circumstances. Regional anaesthetic techniques are also used on the ICU, particularly epidural analgesia using a combination of a low concentration of local anaesthetic and opioids. This technique is suitable for pain relief following surgery or trauma to the thorax, abdomen, pelvis and lower limbs. The incidence of respiratory complications in unventilated patients is reduced as patients are able to take deep breaths and cough forcefully, uninhibited by pain or the respiratory depressant effects of opioids. It is often easier to wean patients off mechanical ventilation using epidural analgesia.

Nutrition

Maintenance of adequate nutrition is an essential element of the care of critically ill patients. Where possible, patients should be fed enterally. *If the gut is working, use it!* Enteral feeding is simpler to administer, less expensive, more physiological and associated with fewer complications than total parenteral nutrition (TPN)(e.g. central line sepsis, acute gastric erosions, hyperglycaemia and specific mineral or vitamin deficiencies). Indications for TPN are listed in Table 9.12.

INDICATION FOR TOTAL PARENTERAL NUTRITION

Ileus following major bowel surgery
Acute pancreatitis
Inflammatory bowel disease
Short bowel syndromes
Malabsorption syndromes
Multiple organ failure
Postoesophagectomy
Severe catabolic states, e.g. extensive burns, sepsis, trauma

Table 9.12 Indication for total parenteral nutrition.

Critically ill patients are at risk of developing acute erosion and ulceration of the gastric mucosa, particularly those who are unable to tolerate enteral feeding leading to the unopposed action of gastric acid. The most appropriate method of ulcer prophylaxis is therefore to provide enteral nutrition at the earliest opportunity. Gastric mucosal protection agents (e.g. sucralfate), which provide prophylaxis against gastric ulceration whilst maintaining the acid environment, are widely used when enteral feeding is not possible.

Infection control

Hospital acquired (nosocomial) infections are associated with increased morbidity and mortality. Critically ill patients on the ICU have a number of risk factors (Table 9.13). Common infections involve the lower respira-

RISK FACTORS FOR NOSOCOMIAL INFECTION

Extremes of age
Pre-existing medical conditions
Poor nutritional status
Immunosuppressive effect of illness, drugs
ICU is a breeding site for antibiotic resistant strains of bacteria
Breach of body surface defences:
    tracheal intubation
    urinary catheter
    i.v. and arterial lines
Raised intragastric pH due to H_2-antagonists

Table 9.13 Risk factors for nosocomial infection on the intensive care unit (ICU).

PREVENTION OF NOSOCOMIAL INFECTION

Good basic hygiene standards, i.e. scrupulous washing of hands immediately before
and after contact with patient, wearing of gloves and aprons
Optimize nutritional status of patient
Avoid overuse of 'prophylactic' broad-spectrum antibiotics
Regular disinfection of ventilator tubing or use of disposable equipment
Use of bacterial/viral filters between patient and ventilator
Insertion of i.v. lines, catheters under full asepsis
Regular toileting of patient, particularly surgical wounds and sites of insertion of i.v.
lines, catheters
Routine changing of i.v. and arterial lines after a defined period (not proven to be
effective)

Table 9.14 Prevention of nosocomial infection on the intensive care unit (ICU).

tory tract in ventilated patients, septicaemia associated with i.v. and arterial lines, and surgical wound infections. Prevention of nosocomial infection should be a priority (Table 9.14). The single most important aspect of prevention is the practice of good hygiene standards.

Common conditions treated on the intensive care unit

RESPIRATORY FAILURE

The causes of respiratory failure and the principles of mechanical ventilation have already been discussed. The most important therapy is oxygen—a life-saving 'drug' and it must be administered in sufficient concentration to raise the Pao_2 to an acceptable level, usually >80 mmHg (10.5 kPa). The severely hypoxic patient who is breathing spontaneously should always be given 100% oxygen by facemask. Unfortunately, many patients are denied high-flow oxygen therapy, inappropriately due to concern that their respiration is dependent on a hypoxic drive. It is not unusual to find young patients with acute severe asthma receiving 28% oxygen because of such fears. Only a minority of patients with chronic obstructive airways disease (blue bloaters) *may* be dependent on a hypoxic ventilatory drive and these patients should have their oxygen therapy carefully titrated. However, even these patients may have 100% oxygen administered as long as their response is carefully observed, clinically and with the aid of arterial blood gas analysis. It is important to remember that it is the partial pressure of oxygen in arterial blood (Pao_2) that is responsible for their respiratory drive, *not* the inspired oxygen concentration.

Although oxygen toxicity occurs when oxygen is administered in high concentration, an inspired concentration $\leq 40\%$ is considered safe for prolonged administration, but it is not logical to withhold higher concentrations in patients with severe respiratory disease.

Appropriate antibiotics should be given in the presence of a chest infection. It is important to obtain a specimen of sputum for microbiological examination and antibiotic-sensitivity testing. Bronchodilators may be useful in patients with bronchospasm associated with asthma or chronic obstructive airways disease, chest infection, pulmonary aspiration or ARDS. Bronchodilators are commonly administered as a nebulized mist directly to the respiratory tract (e.g. salbutamol, ipratropium). They may also be given by i.v. infusion (salbutamol, adrenaline, aminophyline), although there is a greater risk of dysrhythmias. Effective physiotherapy is an essential part of care for all patients in the ICU. Techniques used by physiotherapists in helping to expectorate secretions from the lungs include the positioning of patients to facilitate postural drainage of secretions and percussion of the chest to help loosening of secretions. In those patients being mechanically ventilated, suctioning of the trachea and upper airways is important as many patients, whether paralysed or not, cannot cough effectively. Again, this should be carried out by those trained to do it effectively and safely.

CARDIOVASCULAR FAILURE

The principles of treatment of cardiovascular failure are:

1 to optimize conditions for the left ventricle in order to achieve an appropriate cardiac output and hence oxygen delivery;

2 to optimize the state of the circulatory system such that the cardiac output is distributed to vital organs and tissues at a sufficient pressure for the capillary beds to be well perfused.

This is achieved by correcting hypovolaemia to provide an adequate preload for the left ventricle so that it is functioning at the peak of the Frank–Starling curve (see Fig. 5.2). Any dysrhythmia affecting cardiac performance should be treated. The most common dysrhythmia in patients on the ICU is atrial fibrillation. This not infrequently resolves spontaneously when the patient is adequately fluid resuscitated. Myocardial ischaemia, or the negative inotropic effects of circulating toxic mediators, will reduce myocardial contractility and an inotropic agent may be required, monitored using a PAFC. If sepsis is present, the mean arterial blood pressure may be inadequate in spite of an elevated cardiac output; in this situation a vasoconstrictor is necessary, for example noradrenaline. Vasodilators are used to 'offload' a failing left ventricle. Either strategy requires invasive monitoring of the cardiovascular system.

ACUTE RENAL FAILURE

Critically ill patients with multiple organ failure have significantly different requirements in terms of renal support than do patients with isolated acute or chronic renal failure. An inherently unstable cardiovascular system, the need for large volumes of fluid and the use of potent inotropic and vasoactive drugs mean that these patients are unable to tolerate the relatively rapid fluid and ionic shifts associated with intermittent haemodialysis techniques, which may precipitate cardiovascular collapse. Peritoneal dialysis is also of limited value in the ICU as it does not have the capacity to maintain homeostasis in hypermetabolic patients or remove fluid rapidly enough when required. In addition, it is often not practical in patients following abdominal surgery and with abdominal sepsis. Therefore, to cope with the problems faced by the ICU patient, continuous haemofiltration (analogous to the non-specific filtration that occurs naturally in the glomeruli of the kidneys) is frequently used. An extracorporeal circulation is set up, containing a filter with a semipermeable membrane. Initially, flow through the filter was driven by the patient's own blood pressure (continuous arteriovenous haemofiltration, CAVH). It is now more usual to employ venovenous haemofiltration (CVVH) driven by a roller pump.

SEPSIS SYNDROME

This is a clinical condition in which the host is overwhelmed by an infecting organism producing endotoxin and/or exotoxins. Exotoxins are bacterial products that may be released into the circulation, whereas bacterial endotoxin is a lipopolysaccharide component of the cell membrane of Gram-negative organisms. The majority of infections are endogenous and follow colonization of the alimentary tract by an overgrowth of Gram-negative bacteria that are normally resident, for example *Escherichia coli*, *Klebsiella*, *Proteus* and *Pseudomonas aeruginosa*. Gram-positive staphylococci and streptococci, and fungal infections, particularly candidiasis, may also be implicated. ICU patients are vulnerable either as a result of being immunocompromised or due to their local defence mechanisms being inoperative or bypassed.

The principles of treating sepsis syndrome are the provision of support for failing organ systems (mechanical ventilation, inotropic drugs, fluid resuscitation, haemofiltration, clotting factors, etc.), and targeting the causative organism with appropriate antibiotic therapy. This may require repeated blood cultures and analysis of specimens of sputum, urine, wound and catheter sites to identify the organism responsible. If intra-abdominal pus is a clinical possibility, it must be sought aggressively using ultrasound scanning, computerized tomography (CT) scan or laparotomy. Such patients do *not* recover if surgical drainage is not undertaken. Although haemofiltration is often required due to acute renal failure, there is some evidence that haemofiltration itself may be beneficial to the primary condition by 'filtering out' toxic mediators such as cytokines. In recent years, there have been studies examining the efficacy of monoclonal antibodies to one of the principle cytokines, tumour necrosis factor (TNF), and it is likely that significant advances in the treatment of sepsis syndrome will be made in this area.

Further reading

Andreyev HJ, Forbes A. Parenteral nutrition in adult intensive care. *Postgraduate Medical Journal* 1993; **69**: 841–5.

Beal AL, Cerra FB. Multiple organ failure syndrome in the 1990s. Systemic inflammatory response and organ dysfunction. *Journal of the American Medical Association* 1994; **271**: 226–33.

Edwards JD. Management of septic shock. *British Medical Journal* 1993; **306**: 1661–4.

Hagland MR. The management of acute renal failure in the intensive therapy unit. *Intensive and Critical Care Nursing* 1993; **9**: 237–41.

Kollef MH, Schuster DP. The acute respiratory distress syndrome. *New England Journal of Medicine* 1995; **332**: 27–37.

Oh TE. *Intensive Care Manual*, 3rd edn. London: Butterworths, 1990.

Sproat LJ, Inglis TJJ. Preventing infection in the intensive care unit. *British Journal of Intensive Care* 1992; **2**: 275–85.

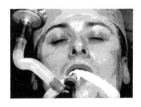

Anaesthetists and Chronic Pain Relief

Anaesthesia is concerned with reducing sensations during surgery; it does not in itself cure patients but enables important treatment to take place without the experience of painful surgery. This is achieved by the application of clinical physiology, pharmacology and therapeutics, as well as nerve blocks. With this expertise in pain and symptom control, some anaesthetists have specialized in the management of pain as a problem in its own right. This has led to the establishment of modern pain relief clinics, which involve a team of anaesthetists, nurses, physiotherapists and psychologists.

THE DEFINITION OF PAIN

The International Association for the Study of Pain defines pain as 'An unpleasant sensory and emotional experience associated with actual or potential tissue damage or described in terms of such damage'.

The complexity of pain

Pain experience may be expressed as written statements, verbal descriptions, facial expressions and other body language.

The experience of pain is the result of many interactions within the central nervous system; previous experiences and present emotional state will determine the reactions to stimuli. The following are examples of this.

• *Effect of changed environment.* For example, a hospital admission where further painful treatment is expected may result in an apparently minor stimulation such as a change of dressing, which may otherwise be tolerated, initiating an overwhelming state of distress.

169

- *Distraction.* A kick on the shin during a game of football is likely to provoke very different pain behaviour when possession is maintained with a clear shot at goal compared to losing a tackle and with it the chance of victory!
- *The meaning of pain.* In the previous example, the football injury and the sensations which we assume to go with it will have a positive meaning. A display of pain behaviour may bring about a reward particularly for a foul in the penalty area. Similar sensations in a cancer patient with a bone metastasis in the tibia may provoke anxiety and fear of pain as yet another problem with no certain end—certainly a negative meaning.
- *The significance of pain.* The symptoms of headache, photophobia and vomiting in a medical student would normally result in presentation at the local casualty department with a diagnosis of meningitis. Exactly the same symptoms would be ignored in the knowledge that he (or she) had drunk 10 pints of lager the night before! Thus pain behaviour is conditioned by knowledge and understanding.
- *The memory and culture of pain.* Pain may leave a memory which will discourage repeating an action, or a response may be learned from observing the behaviour and attitudes of others. This can have both beneficial and detrimental effects.

Cultural differences are important when treating patients of different nationality and race. Age is important: children may not have the means to understand or express pain and simply cry without apparent cause, whereas the elderly may be too ashamed to admit to needing help with pain.

ACUTE AND CHRONIC PAIN

Pain has developed as part of the behaviour keeping us from harm. A hand held against a hot surface is rapidly withdrawn, restricting the thermal damage to the skin. A painful blister on the heel when wearing new shoes is a warning in an attempt to prevent more severe damage to the skin. A healing wound is guarded, preventing stress on newly formed connective tissue and the risk of wound breakdown and a fractured bone is held immobile to allow healing. Pains such as these are referred to as *acute.*

When injury has taken place, pain normally limits activity and promotes healing. The region of the body surrounding the injury may also undergo change, becoming sensitive to even minor stimulation. These changes are known as:

- *hyperaesthesia*—increased appreciation of any stimulus;
- *hyperalgesia*—more intense appreciation of a painful stimulus;
- *allodynia* — sensation of pain in response to a normally non-painful stimulus.

They are mediated partly by locally released substances in the tissues (inflammation), but also by changes in the spinal cord processing of neuronal information. Hyperaesthesia, hyperalgesia and allodynia usually resolve as injuries heal.

Chronic pain suggests persistence of the pain for a long time. There are several useful subdivisions for chronic pain.

1   *Pain from continuing tissue damage.* Arthritis pain is an example of this. Pain usually restricts movement and is useful to prevent further damage to the joints. In contrast, neuropathic joints (i.e. those which have lost sensation) degenerate rapidly.

2   *Cancer pain.* This is usually included as a chronic pain but it is often a combination of several pains from destructive effects of the tumour. Once established, even with treatment, pain is usually a feature of remaining life.

3   *Chronic benign pain—pain despite tissue healing.* The hyperaesthesia and allodynia of acute injury may not resolve with healing of the tissues. This may lead to confusion for both doctors and patients, with repeated attempts at surgical intervention which only exacerbate the problem (e.g. postsurgical back pain does not usually respond to further operations).

4   *Pain without injury.* If hyperaesthesia and allodynia occur for reasons other than injury, a similar pain state will result as when injury is responsible. We do not understand how or why this happens. Apparently trivial stimuli, such as sitting in a cold draught, can produce long-lasting muscle pains without any evidence of tissue injury.

We live in a society with high expectations of medical intervention for injury and illness. Severe pain normally elicits sympathy and naturally we strive to relieve it whenever possible. Prolonged illness or distress results in emotional changes, particularly depression of mood. The failure to recognize that severe pain experience occurs without gross organic pathology and has little relationship to signs of physical disease, exacerbates depression in patients with chronic pain.

The remainder of this chapter considers the understanding, mechanisms and management of the pain problems seen in pain relief clinics.

Mechanisms of pain generation

Although the following account separates the mechanisms of pain generation into distinct entities, there is considerable overlap and interaction. Not only is the experience of pain complex, its generation is also as shown in Fig. 10.1:

A   *Simple stimulation.* Normal activity causing stimulation of tissues can lead to pain, for example the sensation of pressure on the buttocks when sitting for long periods is immediately relieved on shifting position or

MECHANISMS OF PAIN GENERATION

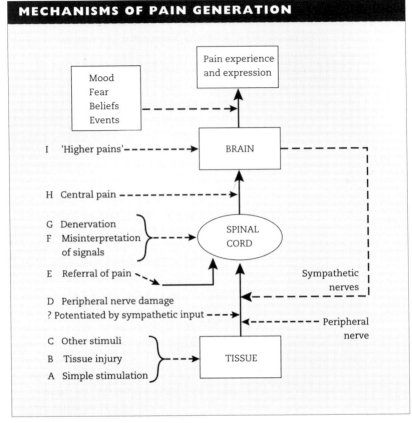

Fig. 10.1 Mechanisms of pain generation.

standing. It is often subconscious and protects us from damage when attention may be focused elsewhere.

B   *Tissue injury.* This results in structural elements being damaged and an inflammatory response occurs. Many chemicals are released including:

- histamine;
- bradykinin;
- 5-hydroxytriptamine (5-HT);
- hydrogen and potassium ions.

Prostaglandins sensitize nerve endings to react more intensely to further stimulation, for example a fingernail when hit with a hammer, although perhaps not showing signs of damage, is very sensitive to further touch and movement.

C   *Other stimuli.* Impulses from pain and temperature receptors are carried in similar small nerve fibres and the threshold for stimulation may be reduced at low temperatures. For example, arthritis patients commonly complain of increased pain during cold weather.

It is not necessary for there to be tissue damage to elicit pain from the periphery, pathways may be stimulated by unusual stimuli; eating ice-cream too quickly often provokes an intense headache but is not perceived as a threat to bodily integrity.

D   *Peripheral nerve damage.* Damage to the nerves supplying an area of the body may result in pain. Peripheral nerves are not normally sensitive to mechanical stimuli, but attempts at regeneration within a damaged nerve may result in a neuroma which can be exquisitely tender. The pain will be referred to the area served by the nerve, although obviously there is no damage to the painful area.

E   *Referred pain.* Pain may be referred from one part of the body to another, for example myocardial ischaemia may present as left-arm or neck pain because the myocardium shares the same cervical segmental innervation.

F   *Misinterpretation of information.* Light touch and pressure stimulation may be interpreted as painful if there is abnormal activity of interneurons in the spinal cord. This may become a permanent feature after injury.

G   *Denervation.* Pain may occur even when sensory receptors are absent, for example after amputation. Sensation can be attributed to an area of the body which does not exist because the brain still has a representation of the absent part (e.g. the painful 'phantom limb'). After spinal cord injury, the central nervous system escapes control from the periphery and pain may be one of the sensations which escapes from peripheral control.

H   *Central pain.* Damage of the thalamic pathways which carry nociceptive information can lead to the experience of pain. As with many chronic pains, the problem is within the central nervous system and it rarely responds to conventional analgesia.

I   *Higher pains.* We have probably all suffered grief, perhaps the death of a loved relative or failure in an important examination. We describe this as painful and although the pain cannot be localized to a particular body part, it is nevertheless very real. This pain exists with no physical input to the body.

The pain of a broken heart is no less real than the pain of a broken leg.

We all have the facility to experience excruciating pain from any part of the body and are prevented from this only by the normal functioning of our nervous systems.

Both noxious stimulation and disorders of transmission or perception have identical results — the experience of pain.

THE VARIABILITY OF PAIN

Pain experience and expression can be triggered and conditioned by many factors other than peripheral noxious stimulation. The body is subjected to millions of stimuli each day, most are of no significance or threat and need to be filtered from entering consciousness or producing a response.

The fact that responses to stimulation can vary in intensity according to factors both within and outside the body led to the work of Melzack and Wall in the 1960s. They published a theory of pain involving the concept of 'gate control' of impulses entering the spinal cord (Fig. 10.2).

I   Sensory information from the periphery is carried in large-diameter (touch and vibration) or small-diameter (pain and temperature) nerve fibres.

2   These synapse onto central transmission neurones in the dorsal horn of the spinal cord (the substantia gelatinosa).

3   Onward transmission is modulated by inhibitory neurones which are switched *on by large-fibre input* and *off by small-fibre input.*

This model explains the effect of stimulation-induced analgesia: large-fibre input activating the inhibitory neurones reducing the input from smaller fibres. We are all familiar with this effect when we suffer a minor injury, our instinct is to 'rub it better'. This action stimulates large fibres

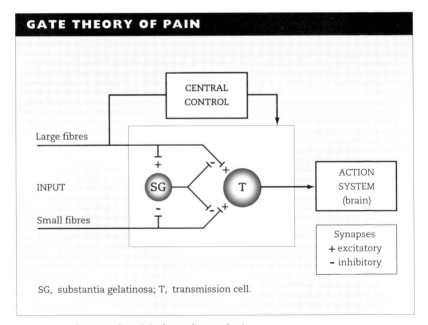

SG, substantia gelatinosa; T, transmission cell.

Fig. 10.2 The original gate theory of pain.

with touch and vibration and reduces the transmission of nociceptive information from small fibres.

The gate control theory is only one example of how the nervous system can modify in response to electrical activity in nerves. The brain also contributes by exerting 'central control' via the descending pathways of the spinal cord, thereby helping to explain how mood and behaviour affect processing within the spinal cord. The whole state is referred to as one of neuroplasticity which occurs in a changing matrix of electrical and neurotransmitter activity rather than a simple fixed electrical circuit.

Clinical assessment of chronic pain

The correct management of the patient with chronic pain is based upon the basic principles of taking a full history and performing a physical examination prior to ordering investigations and initiating treatment.

HISTORY

Site

This may be obvious and related to a previous injury. More diffuse distributions are common. Pain may spread in a dermatomal pattern. Pain may be felt in structures with shared innervation. Pain diagrams are helpful.

Figure 10.3 shows the typical pain distribution resulting from an S1 nerve root compression compared with the pain experience of a patient with fibromyalgia.

Bizarre, so-called 'non-anatomical' pain patterns are common and certainly must not be interpreted as implying that the pain is not genuine.

Character

Some conditions are associated with pain of a particular nature. Lists of words have been used to help patients choose a suitable description (e.g. the McGill pain questionnaire). Trigeminal neuralgia is usually described as shooting and fibromyalgia is described as exhausting, burning and nauseating.

The pain history

Past treatment and investigations are often long and complex, and involve different hospitals and specialists. A complete history will include:

- the time-course of the pain;
- accentuating or relieving factors;
- the pattern of activity and relation to pain;
- the effect on sleep;

PAIN DRAWINGS

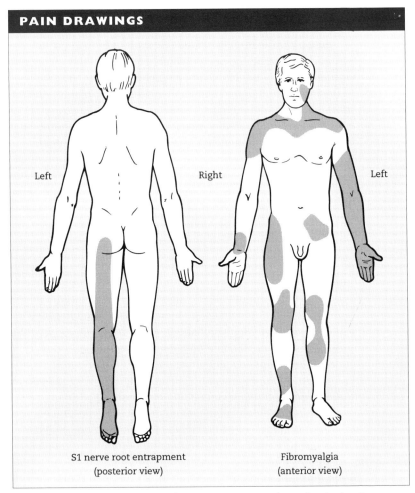

Fig. 10.3 Pain drawings for S1 root entrapment (posterior view) and fibromyalgia (anterior view).

- previous and current treatment including:
  - (a) medication;
  - (b) type and effects of physiotherapy;
  - (c) aids and appliances;
  - (d) alternative therapies tried;
- the effect on employment;
- financial support:
  - (a) invalidity benefits;

(b) pensions;

(c) Disability Living Allowance, etc.;

- social and family losses because of pain;
- concerns about the future;
- uncertainties about diagnosis and treatment;
- past medical history, including episodes of vague or unexplained illnesses;
- family history may reveal clues as to coping mechanisms and attitude to chronic illness within the family.

> A most helpful question to ask the patient is what they think is causing the pain.

Psychological assessment

An assessment of mood is important and frequently reveals evidence of depression. This may be related to the pain itself, but is also associated with frustration at many previous attempts at treatment or the failure of treatment, lack of a clear diagnosis or disease, and loss of social and financial status. These are all commonly associated with chronic pain. The assistance of a psychologist is invaluable to explore emotional issues associated with, or caused by, the pain.

Patients should, wherever possible, be seen with a spouse to assess independently the degree of physical and emotional disturbance in the home.

PHYSICAL EXAMINATION

It is unusual for patients to present with 'put on' symptoms of pain. Malingering is very rare. Often symptoms and the reaction to examination are exaggerated, but this is not surprising considering that most patients with years of suffering are likely to be distressed and anxious. Most patients experience worse pain after even limited clinical examination.

Pain may be associated with the following structures:

- *bones:* deformity, tenderness;
- *joints:* swelling, tenderness, limitation of movement;
- *nerves:* function, swelling or tenderness over the course of a peripheral nerve;
- *muscles:* power and tone, localized or generalized tenderness;
- *skin:* signs of sympathetic dysfunction:
  (a) temperature change;
  (b) loss of hair growth;

(c) vascular changes and discoloration;

(d) disorders of sensation.

In addition, loss of confidence in movements, guarding and abnormal posture are noted as possible contributions to maintaining chronic pain.

MEASUREMENT OF PAIN

Useful information may be obtained by measuring the effects of the pain and how, or if, life would be different without pain. This can be done using simple numerical or linear analogue scales or a 'pain thermometer'. Psychological measures of coping, distress and depression are all useful tools in exploring the pain and should be conducted in conjunction with the clinical psychologist.

INVESTIGATIONS

Patients with chronic pain have usually had many investigations. Care must be taken to explain that the absence of positive findings does not mean that the pain is in any way 'imaginary', 'all in the mind' or 'psychological'. One danger of sensitive tests, such as nuclear magnetic resonance scanning, is that abnormalities which are coincidental to the pain may be revealed.

TREATMENT

There are very few effective 'cures' for chronic pain problems. A positive attitude to intervention is only appropriate if there is a realistic chance of success — an honest opinion is appreciated. For some conditions associated with ongoing tissue damage, such as rheumatoid arthritis, it is possible to suppress the inflammation and the associated pain. This may not be completely successful, as the treatment of pain may have to proceed alongside treatment of the condition.

Pharmacological management (Fig. 10.4)

OPIOIDS (see also page 71)

Morphine is commonly used in the management of acute pain and has a major role in control of chronic pain although its prescription is significantly different. The oral route is widely used, often starting at 10 mg every 4 hours, with as much as 1000 mg per 24 hours required in some conditions. The daily dose may be given as a long-acting sustained-release preparation twice a day. Respiratory depression (often a feared complication) is *not* seen, even with very high doses, provided that doses are increased in a logical fashion — usually by 50% increments every 3 days.

SITES OF ACTION OF ANALGESIC DRUGS

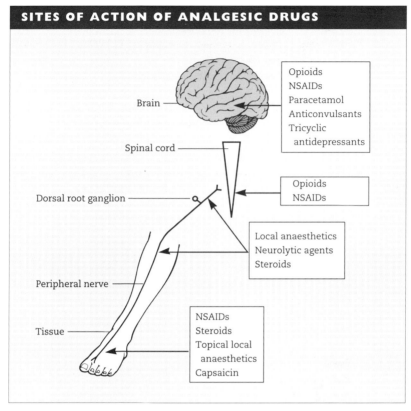

Fig. 10.4 Sites of action of analgesic drugs.

Sedation may predispose to pneumonia and shorten life. This must be balanced against the humanitarian benefits of symptom control. Alternatives are diamorphine, which is often used for subcutaneous infusions as it is very soluble and can be dissolved in a small volume for administration using a compact pump, and methadone which has a long plasma half-life and may be given as a once daily dose orally.

Weaker opioids such as dextropropoxyphene (combined with paracetamol in coproxamol) and codeine or dihydrocodeine are commonly prescribed as tablets for chronic pain. They have the same effects and side-effects as morphine but the maximum analgesia is limited.

NON-STEROIDAL ANTI-INFLAMMATORY DRUGS

Non-steroidal anti-inflammatory drugs (NSAIDs) are often used alone or in combination with opioids, particularly where there is an element of bone pain. Their mechanism of action and side-effects are discussed on page 77. Many are available, but the most widely known is aspirin. For longer term use, ibuprofen, naproxen or diclofenac may produce fewer side-effects. Gastric effects may be reduced by H_2-antagonists, prostaglandin analogues, or antacid medications.

TRICYCLIC ANTIDEPRESSANTS

The mechanism of this group of drugs is thought to be due to central monoamine and cholinergic effects. Amitriptyline is the most commonly used drug, and has been used extensively to treat neuropathic pain. The sedative effect may be useful for sleep disturbance if given at night. The antidepressant effect may be useful when depression requires therapy. Newer antidepressants with fewer side-effects offer no advantage in the management of pain.

ANTICONVULSANTS

Trigeminal neuralgia (TGN) is a brief, recurrent, stabbing pain in the distribution of one or more branches of the fifth cranial nerve. It responds particularly well to carbamazepine or phenytoin (although surgical decompression or destructive lesions of the trigeminal ganglion are also effective).

STIMULANTS

Caffeine is a constituent of some migraine preparations. It may have analgesic properties by central effects. Dexamphetamine has also been used both as an analgesic and to reverse the sedative effects of large doses of morphine in terminal illness.

STEROIDS

These may be useful to reduce swelling and compression from tumours in malignant states. They are not indicated for chronic benign pain because of the risk of osteoporosis and gastric ulceration. Injections of steroid are given in combination with local anaesthetic into the epidural space when nerve roots are thought to be trapped. The benefit may be due to a reduction in nerve root oedema.

CAPSAICIN

Applied topically as a cream, this extract of the red chilli pepper can depress C-fibre nerve function. It has been found useful in postherpetic neuralgia. It produces a burning sensation on first use but if tolerated, regular use may reduce pain symptoms.

TOPICAL LOCAL ANAESTHETICS

Applied over the painful area of skin, very small concentrations may dramatically reduce symptoms without producing numbness.

Non-pharmacological intervention (Fig. 10.5)

NERVE BLOCKS

These may be performed on any nerve which is thought to be involved in pain generation. Where pain is due to disordered central processing (e.g. allodynia), local anaesthetic block of nerve input (light touch) may temporarily abolish the pain. Attempts to make blocks permanent with neurolytic agents often result in worse pain as central neurones become increasingly sensitive and responsive to previously non-painful stimuli.

The spinothalamic tracts carry nociceptive information from the contralateral side of the body and may be interrupted at the level of the cervical spine by a cordotomy (cutting the cord) performed surgically at open operation or percutaneously with a radiofrequency lesion-generating needle.

STIMULATION

Stimulation of the nervous system appears to be an effective method of decreasing some pains. Massage may be helpful, but more specifically, electrical stimulation using electrodes on the skin (transcutaneous nerve stimulation, TENS), or in the epidural space (spinal cord stimulation) may produce benefit. Acupuncture involves identifying and needling specific points on the body surface according to patterns determined by traditional Chinese medical practice.

MANIPULATION

Osteopathy and chiropractic techniques are practised widely for chronic musculoskeletal pain. Mobilization certainly has an important role, but these techniques have not been satisfactorily compared with current medical rehabilitation procedures.

PHYSIOTHERAPY

Physiotherapists are able to perform assessments of physical structure and function. Posture, gait and function often become abnormal as a result of chronic pain. Confidence needs to be rebuilt.

OTHER METHODS OF PROVIDING ANALGESIA

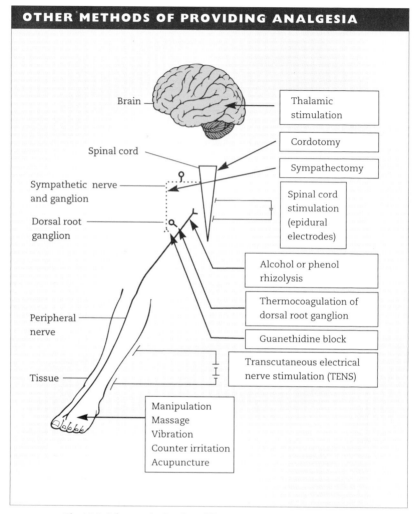

Fig. 10.5 Other methods of providing analgesia.

PSYCHOLOGY

It is unusual for patients to present with chronic pain without distress or depression. This is often as a result of the frustration of limited activity and many failed attempts at treatment. Psychologists are essential in helping to overcome these problems.

Common chronic pain problems

POSTOPERATIVE PAIN

Although usually acute and self-limiting, postoperative pain may progress to chronic pain. Nerve damage is the most frequent association, for example post-thoracotomy intercostal nerve damage or ilio-inguinal nerve damage from inguinal hernia repair. Both are persistent and troublesome, nerve block may be helpful diagnostically but proceeding to neurolytic block does not give lasting benefit.

CANCER PAIN

Cancers involving destruction of tissue are painful. Two-thirds of patients with cancer as a terminal illness have significant pain. Modern chemotherapy, radiotherapy and surgery can reduce the growth of tumour, but pain may persist even despite technically successful therapy. Pain may be feared more than death itself. Symptoms can become overwhelming—a mixture of pain, fear, depression, panic and denial — the so-called 'total pain syndrome'.

Morphine is not available for clinical use in many developing countries. Even in western countries, use is inadequate due to fear of side-effects. Large doses of morphine may be required (compared to those used to treat acute pain), but when correctly used it is safe and effective for most cancer pain.

NEUROPATHIC PAIN

Postherpetic neuralgia

Postherpetic neuralgia (PHN) is a common consequence of infection with the herpes zoster virus, with damage to the sensory nerve cells in the dorsal root ganglion. The painful crusted lesions on the skin (on the corresponding dermatome to the infected nerve) heal after several weeks but the site often has persistent abnormal sensation, with light touch producing pain (allodynia).

Antiviral agents, topically or systemically during the initial infection, may limit nerve damage and subsequent neuralgia and early sympathetic blocks may be of benefit, for example stellate ganglion or lumbar sympathetic blocks.

Sympathetically maintained pain

Nerves in damaged tissues appear to be particularly sensitive to sympathetic stimulation (noradrenaline released from the nerve endings).

Sometimes a well-defined syndrome develops as a result of injury, consisting of redness, swelling, burning pain with shiny hairless skin. Originally called reflex sympathetic dystrophy, it is now included in complex regional pain syndrome. Occasionally no cause or triggering event can be identified.

It may respond to sympathetic denervation, either by nerve block of the ganglia (cervical or lumbar, temporary or neurolytic) or by local infusion of guanethidine which depletes sympathetic nerve cells of noradrenaline. Some other types of neuropathic pain also respond to sympathectomy.

Arthritis

In this debilitating condition, pain is a frequent symptom of joint inflammation and destruction. Most patients are managed by general practitioners or by rheumatologists. Patients with severe arthritis have visible deformity and disability, which leads to their suffering and pain being understood by others and is often well tolerated. NSAIDs and opioids are usually effective when used in addition to specific therapy for the disease.

Back pain

More than half the population will suffer back pain at some time in their lives. With advancing age, spinal degenerative changes are common, but these changes do not correlate with back pain symptoms. Unfortunately, treatment is not available for most degenerative changes — there is little evidence that replacing worn discs or fusing spinal segments has long-term beneficial effects. Most important is early exclusion of specific causes of back pain. These are:

• prolapsed intervertebral disc with spinal cord or nerve root compression;
• tumour of bone, meninges or nerves;
• infection of the spine.

New episodes of back pain should be appropriately investigated and the patient reassured. Early mobilization and activity is important to prevent dysfunction and guarding of movements of the back. Even 2 days of bed rest may be harmful. Most patients are given advice to rest until the pain subsides, and investigation is undertaken only after a long delay. This leads to unnecessary suffering and dissatisfaction with the medical profession. Treatment involves acknowledging the pain, education, gradual return to activity under strict supervision and the introduction of coping skills for pain.

The chronic pain syndrome

The precise cause and mechanism of much pain is not known. Many chronic-pain clinic patients have the following characteristics:

- a long history;
- many consultations;
- multiple negative investigations;
- a high incidence of functional disturbance, for example headache, irritable bowel syndrome;
- few standard physical findings;
- distress;
- depression.

Medicolegal proceedings are common but only rarely result in deliberate exaggeration of symptoms. The medical examination of these patients requires experience and understanding of the context in which the pain is being experienced. Even experienced clinicians have been known to accuse these patients of malingering.

Patients may have coped well with the pain for a long period of time—it is usually a series of events as a consequence of the pain which precipitates referral. Measures aimed at dealing with the pain may be useless if, for example, the patient has become depressed, is dependent on medication, has lost their employment and self respect, and been accused of malingering. Treatment is aimed at coping with pain, which in turn depends on:

- understanding that chronic pain is harmless (but painful);
- stopping looking for a cure;
- accepting some limitations;
- knowledge that nothing is being hidden;
- willingness to change (effort required).

PREVENTING CHRONIC PAIN

It may be possible to prevent chronic pain by more aggressive treatment of acute pain. Identification of risk factors, early education and discussion may help to prevent loss of function and the frustration which often lead to chronic pain.

Further reading

Bonica JJ. *The Management of Pain*, 2nd edn. Pennsylvania, USA: Lea Febiger, 1990.
Melzack R, Wall PD. *The Challenge of Pain*. London: Penguin, 1988.

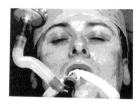

Resuscitation of the Collapsed Patient

The resuscitation of a collapsed patient is usually divided into two phases.
I *Basic life support (BLS)* is the description given to the technique of maintaining the airway, breathing and circulation without the use of any equipment. The use of simple protective shields interposed between the mouth of the rescuer and patient is allowed (e.g. Laerdal pocket mask). BLS is performed to limit hypoxic damage of the vital organs by providing an artificial circulation; it rarely results in the return of a spontaneous circulation, but is essential to maximize the chances of advanced life support achieving this.
2 *Advanced life support (ALS)* is the description given to the use of defibrillation, intubation and the administration of drugs in an attempt to restore a spontaneous circulation as this maximizes a patient's chances of recovery.

The aims of this chapter are to provide an outline of the techniques used in BLS and ALS which are not covered elsewhere in the book. The reader should consult the current Resuscitation Council (UK) guidelines for details of how these techniques are integrated into management algorithms.

Adult basic life support

In order that the rescuer suffers no harm, and that BLS is carried out appropriately and in the most efficient manner, the following sequence of actions should be performed.

The SAFE approach
I *Shout for help.* BLS is physically demanding and is more effectively performed by two rescuers. The arrival of any help allows summoning of advanced help via a telephone.

186

2   *Approach a collapsed person with care.* Never putting oneself (or others) at risk. This is clearly important when the collapse occurs outside of the hospital environment, where there may be gas, toxic fumes, traffic, electricity or fire, endangering the rescuer or patient.

3   *Free both the victim and rescuer from danger before commencing resuscitation.* If it is perceived that there are risks to either the victim or rescuers, then the patient must be moved to a place of greater safety.

4   *Evaluate the patient.* Not all collapsed patients will need (or appreciate) artificial ventilation and external cardiac compressions.

Patient evaluation

The first step is to see if the patient is responsive, by placing one hand on the patient's forehead, shaking the shoulders gently with the other hand whilst at the same time asking loudly 'Are you all right?'

Points to note

• The head is held stable during the assessment to guard against the possibility of aggravating an injury to the cervical spine.

• Always assume the patient might be deaf, therefore ensure he/she can see your lips move when assessing responsiveness.

• In the responsive patient, where there is obvious trauma, immobilize the cervical spine by in-line stabilization until help arrives (Fig. 11.1).

Airway control

In most unconscious patients, the airway will become obstructed. This occurs most often at the level of the hypopharynx as the reduced tone in the muscles of the tongue, jaw and neck allow the tongue to fall

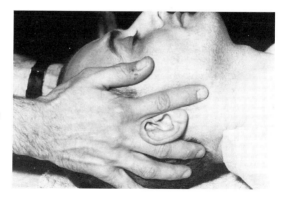

Fig. 11.1 In-line cervical stabilization. Note position of index finger maintaining a slight jaw thrust. Courtesy of Greaves I, Hodgetts T, Porter K. *Emergency Care—A Textbook for Paramedics.* London: Harcourt Brace, 1997.

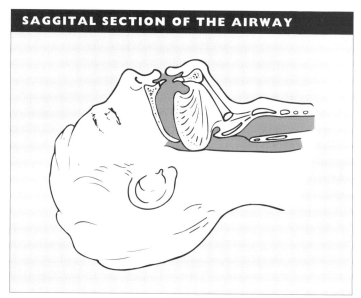

Fig. 11.2 Saggital section of the airway.

against the posterior pharyngeal wall (Fig. 11.2). Correction, using the following techniques, may allow recovery without the need for further intervention.

• *Head tilt plus chin lift* (Fig. 11.3). The rescuer's hand nearest the head is placed on the forehead, gently extending the head backwards. The chin is then lifted using the index and middle fingers of the rescuer's other hand. If the mouth closes, the lower lip should be retracted downwards by the thumb.

• *Jaw thrust* (Fig. 11.4). This is used if the above technique fails to create an airway, or there is a suspicion that the cervical spine may have been injured. The patient's jaw is 'thrust' upwards (forwards) by applying pressure behind the angles of the mandible, either by the rescuer using their thumbs or alternatively their fingertips. This manoeuvre is often combined with a head tilt and the tips of the thumbs are used to open the mouth, and it is referred to as the 'triple airway manoeuvre'.

• *Finger sweep*. The mouth must be opened and inspected, and any obvious material contributing to the obstruction removed by placing a finger in the mouth and gently sweeping from side to back, 'hooking' out loose material. At the same time, broken, loose or partial dentures should be removed, but well-fitting ones may be left in place (see later).

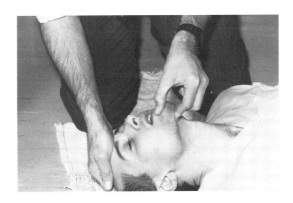

Fig. 11.3 Head tilt, chin lift. Courtesy of Greaves I, Hodgetts T, Porter K. *Emergency Care—A Textbook for Paramedics*. London: Harcourt Brace, 1997.

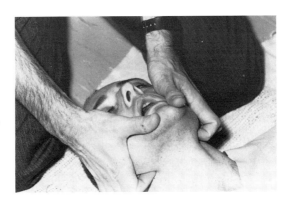

Fig. 11.4 Triple manoeuvre. Courtesy of Greaves I, Hodgetts T, Porter K. *Emergency Care—A Textbook for Paramedics*. London: Harcourt Brace, 1997.

Breathing

Having created an airway using one of the above techniques, the patient's breathing must now be rapidly evaluated in the following manner (Fig. 11.5).

- *Look:* down the line of the chest to see if it is rising and falling.
- *Listen:* at the mouth and nose for breath sound, gurgling or snoring sounds.
- *Feel:* for expired air at the patient's mouth and nose with the side of one's cheek.

> Look, listen and feel for up to 10 seconds before deciding whether breathing is absent.

If there is no evidence of spontaneous ventilation, then 'mouth-to-mouth' or more correctly expired-air ventilation will be required.

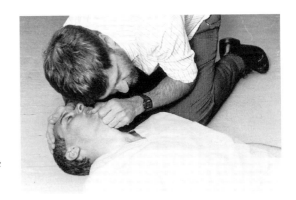

Fig. 11.5 Look, listen, feel.
Courtesy of Greaves I,
Hodgetts T, Porter K.
*Emergency Care—A Textbook
for Paramedics.* London:
Harcourt Brace, 1997.

THE TECHNIQUE OF EXPIRED-AIR VENTILATION

To successfully ventilate a patient with expired air, there must be a clear path, with no leaks, between the rescuer's lungs and the patient's lungs.

Mouth-to-mouth ventilation

1   Keep the patient's airway patent by performing a head tilt and using the index finger and thumb of the same hand to pinch the patient's nose to prevent leaks. The fingers of the lower hand are then used to perform a chin lift, and if necessary open the patient's mouth (Fig. 11.6a).

2   The rescuer takes a deep breath in and makes a seal with their lips around the patient's mouth. Well-fitting dentures are often usefully left *in situ* as they help maintain the contour of the mouth and make it easier to create a good seal.

3   The rescuer then breaths out into the patient's mouth for 1.5–2 seconds, at the same time listening for leaks and looking down the patient's chest to ensure it rises (Fig. 11.6b).

4   Maintaining the head tilt/chin lift, the rescuer now moves away from the mouth to allow passive exhalation for 2–4 seconds, watching to ensure the chest falls (Fig. 11.6c).

Each complete cycle of expired-air ventilation should take 5–6 seconds, thereby allowing 10–12 breaths per minute.

Mouth-to-nose ventilation

This technique is used where mouth-to-mouth ventilation is unsuccessful, for example if an obstruction in the mouth cannot be relieved, or when the rescuer is a child. The airway is maintained as already described, but the mouth is closed with the fingers of the lower hand. The seal is made between the rescuer's lips around the base of the patient's nose.

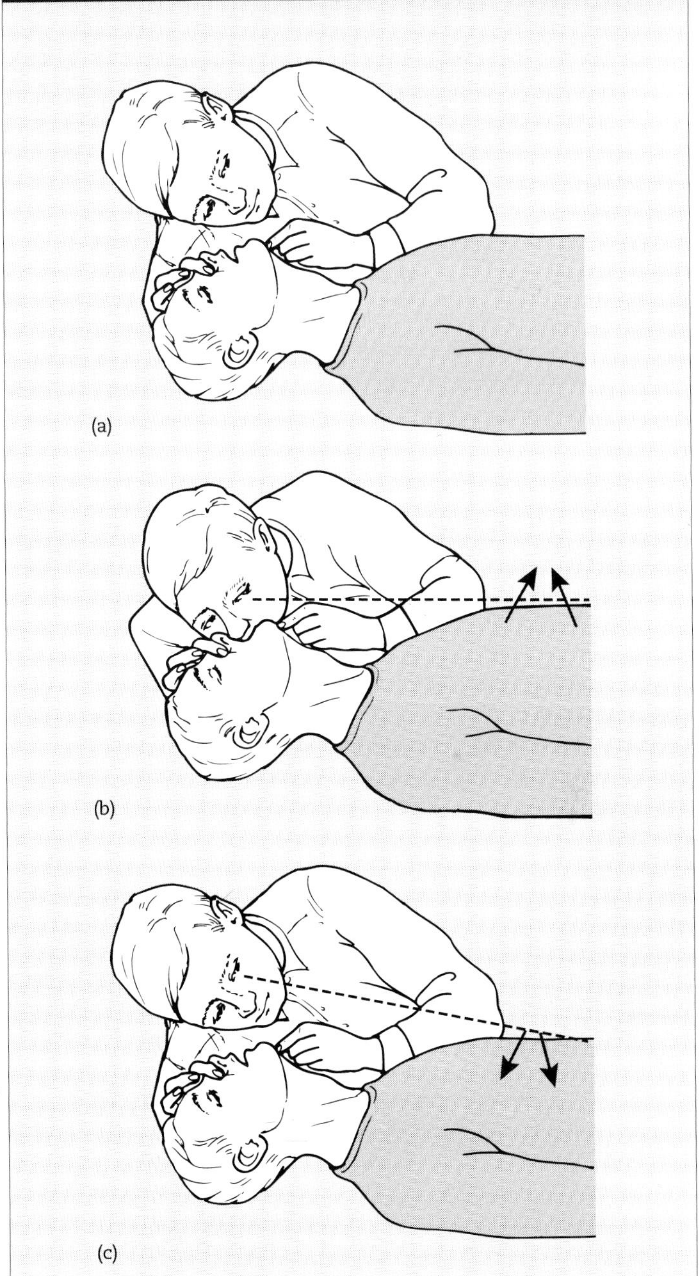

Fig. 11.6 (a–c) Mouth-to-mouth ventilation.

Inspiration is as above, checking to ensure that the chest rises, and the mouth is then opened to assist with expiration, the rescuer watching to ensure that the chest now falls.

> **Common causes of inadequate ventilation**
> - *Obstruction:* failing to maintain head tilt, chin lift.
> - *Leaks:* inadequate seal around the mouth or failure to occlude the patient's nose.
> - *Exhaling too hard:* trying to overcome an obstructed airway, resulting in gastric distension.
> - *Foreign body:* unrecognized in the patient's airway.

Circulation

A check must now be made for evidence of the patient's circulation by feeling for a pulse. In an emergency, central arteries are more reliable than peripheral ones as a pulse will be palpable even with a very low cardiac output. The carotid artery is usually the most accessible and acceptable. If there is no evidence of a spontaneous circulation, external cardiac compression will be required.

THE TECHNIQUE OF EXTERNAL CARDIAC COMPRESSION

This technique only results in a maximum cardiac output 30% of normal, probably by a combination of direct compression of the heart between the sternum and the spine, along with a sudden rise in the intrathoracic pressure during compression. In order to achieve this, the position of the hands is critical.

1 The rescuer positions him/herself on one side of the patient.

2 The patient's chest is exposed and the xiphisternum identified.

3 The index and middle fingers of the rescuer's lower hand are placed on the xiphisternum and the heel of the other hand is placed adjacent to them on the sternum (Fig. 11.7a).

4 The fingers are then removed and the heel of the second hand placed on the back of the hand on the sternum. The fingers may then be interlocked.

5 The sternum is depressed vertically 4–5 cm and then released rapidly. This is repeated at a rate of approximately 100/minute, compression and relaxation each taking the same length of time.

6 To optimize compression and reduce rescuer fatigue chest compressions are best performed with the rescuer leaning well forward over the patient, arms straight and hands, elbows and shoulders extended in a

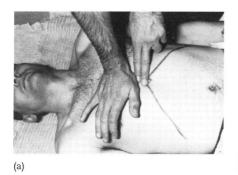

(a)

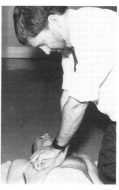

(b)

Fig. 11.7 (a,b) External cardiac compression. Courtesy of Greaves I, Hodgetts T, Porter K. *Emergency Care—A Textbook for Paramedics*. London: Harcourt Brace, 1997.

straight line. This allows use of the rescuer's upper body weight to achieve compression, rather than the arm muscles, which will rapidly tire and reduce efficiency (Fig. 11.7b).

Common causes of inadequate cardiac output

- Wrong hand position:
  (a) too high: the heart is not compressed;
  (b) too low: the stomach is compressed and risk of aspiration increased;
  (c) too laterally: injures underlying organs, for example liver, spleen, bowel.
- Over-enthusiastic effort:
  (a) causes cardiac damage;
  (b) fractures ribs which may damage underlying organs, particularly lungs and liver.
- Inadequate effort:
  (a) the rescuer is not high enough above the patient to use his/her body weight;
  (b) fatigue during prolonged resuscitation or poor technique.
- Failure to release between compressions: prevents venous return and filling of the heart.
- Inadequate or excessive rate:
  (a) <80/minute;
  (b) >100/minute.

If the patient is not breathing and does not have a pulse, this is often referred to as a 'cardiac arrest'. The combination of expired-air ventilation and external cardiac compression will be required and this is frequently referred to as cardiopulmonary resuscitation or CPR.

CARDIOPULMONARY RESUSCITATION

With a single rescuer, two expired-air ventilations are given, followed immediately by 15 external cardiac compressions. This cycle (2:15) is performed continuously, each time tilting the patient's head, lifting the chin to create a patent airway, and checking the correct position of the hands before commencing chest compressions.

With two rescuers, the cycle used is one breath followed by five compressions. This cycle (1:5) is performed continuously, each breath should again last for approximately 1.5–2 seconds, with external cardiac compression stopping momentarily to allow ventilation, then recommencing without waiting for exhalation to occur. Where there are two rescuers, the person performing external cardiac compression can leave their hands on the sternum between each series of compressions, but in doing so the pressure must be totally released so as not to compromise ventilation.

Once commenced, CPR must not be interrupted unless the patient shows signs of spontaneous ventilation or movement. If this does happen, then the carotid pulse should be reassessed for 5 seconds before deciding how to continue. However, such an occurrence is extremely rare.

SUMMONING HELP

BLS alone is unlikely to result in the return of a spontaneous circulation and the best chance of survival is if the heart arrests in ventricular fibrillation (VF) and the skills of ALS (see below) are commenced early. The latter are usually provided along with the appropriate equipment by the emergency services, who have to be summoned by telephone. If more than one person is available to carry out resuscitation, then clearly, one person should be despatched rapidly to alert the emergency services and then return to assist with BLS as necessary.

When there is only a single rescuer, the situation is more difficult. Having discovered a collapsed person, should one start BLS, or leave the victim and telephone the emergency services? As the single most important determinant of survival from VF is the time from collapse to the first attempt at defibrillation, then time should not be wasted starting BLS — telephone for help! On returning to the patient, BLS can then be commenced. Where a telephone is not readily available, for example in open countryside, then a few minutes of BLS may be attempted, but it must be understood that the chances of successful resuscitation are very poor.

BASIC LIFE SUPPORT AND INFECTION RISK

The risk of transmission of infectious diseases from casualties to rescuers during mouth-to-mouth resuscitation is extremely low and there have been no reported cases of transmission of either hepatitis B or human immunodeficiency virus (HIV) through mouth-to-mouth ventilation, with sputum, saliva, sweat and tears all being low-risk fluids. Precautions should be taken, if possible, in cases where there might be contact with blood, particularly if any bodily secretion contains visible blood. In these circumstances, devices are available which prevent direct contact between the rescuer and the victim (such as resuscitation masks). Swabs or any other porous material placed over the victim's mouth are of no benefit in this regard. Although practice manikins have not been shown to be a source of infection, they should be cleaned regularly as recommended in the manufacturer's instructions.

The choking patient

Although almost any foreign body can cause airway obstruction, in adults it is usually food, as a result of trying to eat, talk and breathe simultaneously, termed the 'cafe coronary'. In these circumstances adults show signs of acute airway obstruction with extreme distress and activity to try and dislodge the obstruction. If obstruction is incomplete, there may be severe coughing and inspiratory stridor.

MANAGEMENT

If the victim is still conscious, then back blows should be used initially. Standing to one side of the patient, the rescuer should encourage the patient to lean forwards and while supporting his/her chest with one hand, five firm blows are delivered between the patient's scapulae. If the obstruction is relieved quickly, not all five blows need to be delivered. If this fails, then proceed rapidly to the Heimlich manoeuvre.

THE HEIMLICH MANOEUVRE

This aims to produce a rapid rise in intrathoracic pressure by forcing the diaphragm into the chest, and expel the foreign body. It can be performed with the patient standing, sitting or kneeling down.

In a standing patient:
- the rescuer moves behind the victim, passing both arms around him/her at the level of the upper abdomen;
- the rescuer then makes one hand into a fist and places it firmly in the patient's epigastrium, the rescuer's other hand is then placed over the fist;

- both hands are forced vigorously upwards and backwards into the epigastrium and this is repeated 5–10 times unless the foreign body is dislodged sooner (Fig. 11.8);
- this will force the object into a position where the patient can remove
it by coughing or hooking it out with a finger.

If the patient is unconscious:
- place them in a supine position and quickly attempt a finger sweep;
- the rescuer then kneels astride the patient, facing his/her head;
- the rescuer's hands are placed in the epigastrium in the same way as
described above, and a series of vigorous thrusts applied upwards and
backwards, in the midline;

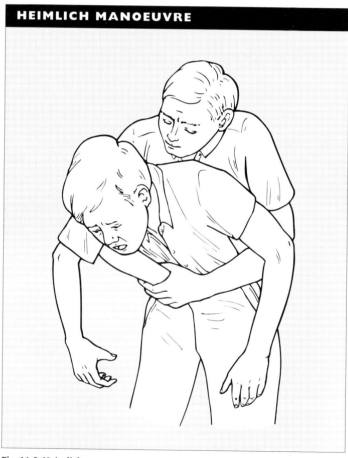

HEIMLICH MANOEUVRE

Fig. 11.8 Heimlich manoeuvre.

- Five to ten thrusts are applied, after which the airway should be inspected and a finger sweep performed to check for any dislodged objects.

If this fails to remove the obstruction, two further series of 10 thrusts can be applied, or alternatively chest thrusts in the style of external cardiac compressions used during CPR can be tried. If these efforts fail to clear the obstruction, little else can be done without equipment for laryngoscopy and intubation or the creation of a surgical airway (cricothyroidotomy; see page 52).

Paediatric basic life support

Paediatric BLS is not a scaled-down version of adult BLS. Although the general principles are the same, specific techniques are required if the optimum support is to be given and the techniques are varied according to the size of the child. 'Infant' is used to mean those less than 1 year old and 'small children' less than 8 years old.

The SAFE approach and evaluation of the patient are as for adults, accepting that infants and very small children who cannot yet talk, and older children who are very scared, are unlikely to reply meaningfully, but they may make some sound or open their eyes to the rescuer's voice.

Airway control

If the child is not breathing it may be because the airway has been blocked by the tongue falling back to obstruct the pharynx. Correction of this problem may result in recovery without further intervention.

- *Head tilt plus chin lift.* A hand is placed on the forehead, the head is gently tilted back as for an adult. In an infant, the tilt should be just sufficient to place the head in a neutral position. The fingers of the other hand should then be placed under the chin, lifting it upwards. Care should be taken not to injure the soft tissue by gripping too hard. It may be necessary to use the thumb of the same hand to part the lips slightly.
- *Jaw thrust.* This is achieved by placing two or three fingers under the angle of the mandible bilaterally, and lifting the jaw upwards. This technique may be easier if the rescuer's elbows are resting on the same surface as the child is lying on. A small degree of head tilt may also be applied.

The finger sweep technique often recommended in adults should not be used in children. The child's soft palate is easily damaged causing bleeding, and foreign bodies may become impacted in the child's cone-shaped airway and be even more difficult to remove.

Breathing

Having created an airway using one of the above techniques, the adequacy of ventilation should then be assessed rapidly in the same manner as for adults, by looking, listening and feeling for up to 10 seconds, and if absent, expired-air ventilation will be required.

THE TECHNIQUE OF EXPIRED-AIR VENTILATION

The airway is kept open using the techniques described above. If the mouth of the child alone is used, then the nose should be pinched closed using the thumb and index fingers of the hand that is maintaining the head tilt. In infants and small children, mouth-to-mouth and nose ventilation should be used.

Since children vary in size, only general guidance can be given regarding the volume and pressure of inflation. This is shown in Table 11.1.

If the chest does not rise then the airway is not clear:
- readjust the head tilt/chin lift position;
- try a jaw thrust;
- if both fail to provide a clear airway, suspect that a foreign body is causing obstruction, and take the appropriate action (see below).

Circulation

In children the carotid artery can be palpated, but in infants the neck is generally short and fat, and it may be difficult to identify. Alternatives are the brachial artery on the medial aspect of the upper arm or the femoral artery.

In children, absence of the circulation is defined as no evidence of a major pulse for 5 seconds, but in infants the circulation is considered inadequate with a heart rate less than 60 beats/minute necessitating external cardiac compression.

THE TECHNIQUE OF EXTERNAL CARDIAC COMPRESSION IN CHILDREN

Children vary in size, and the compressions given should reflect this. In general, infants (< 1 year) require a different technique from small children. In children over 8 years of age, the method used in adults can be applied with appropriate modifications for their size.

GENERAL GUIDANCE

The chest should be seen to rise
Inflation pressure may be higher since airways are small
Slow breaths at the lowest pressure reduce gastric distention

Table 11.1 General guidance for expired air ventilation.

Infants

The infant heart is lower compared to external landmarks, the area of compression is found by imagining a line running between the nipples and compressing over the sternum one finger's breadth below this line. Two fingers are used to compress the chest to a depth of approximately 1.5–2.5 cm (Fig. 11.9).

An alternative in infants is the hand-encircling technique. The infant is held with both the rescuer's hands encircling the chest. The thumbs are placed over the correct part of the sternum (see above) and compression carried out.

Small children

The area of compression is one finger's breadth above the xiphisternum.

INFANT CARDIAC COMPRESSION

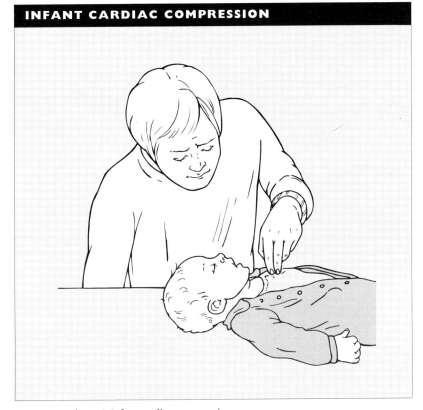

Fig. 11.9 Infant cardiac compression.

CARDIAC COMPRESSION IN A SMALL CHILD

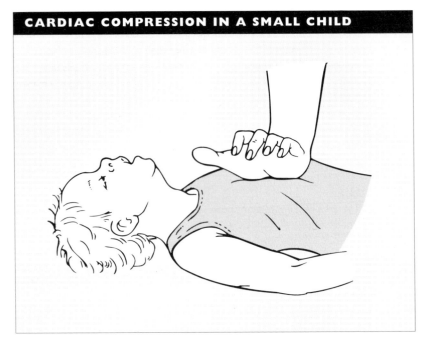

Fig. 11.10 Cardiac compression in a small child.

The heel of one hand is used to compress the sternum to a depth of approximately 2.5–3.5 cm (Fig. 11.10).

Larger children

The area of compression is two fingers' breadth above the xiphisternum. The heels of both hands are used to compress the sternum to a depth of approximately 3–4 cm depending on the size of the child.

Infants and children have a requirement for higher rates of ventilation and compression than adults and the aim should be to complete 20 cycles of one breath followed by five compressions (1:5)/minute. Clearly, time spent readjusting the airway or re-establishing the correct position for compressions will seriously decrease the number of cycles given per minute. This can be a very real problem for the solo rescuer and there is no easy solution. The CPR manoeuvres recommended for infants and children are summarized in Table 11.2.

THE CHOKING CHILD

Foreign body aspiration occurs most commonly in preschool children, who inhale almost anything. The diagnosis should be suspected in any child

CPR IN CHILDREN

	Infant	Small child	Larger child
Airway			
Head tilt position	Neutral	Sniffing	Sniffing
Breathing			
Initial slow breaths	5	5	5
Circulation			
Pulse check	Brachial or femoral	Carotid	Carotid
Landmark	1 finger's breadth below nipple line	1 finger's breadth above xiphisternum	2 fingers' breadth above xiphisternum
Technique	2 fingers or encircling	1 hand	2 hands
Depth	1.5–2.5 cm	2.5–3.5 cm	3–4 cm
CPR			
Ratio	1:5	1:5	1:5
Cycles per minute	20	20	20

Table 11.2 Summary of cardiopulmonary resuscitation (CPR) manoeuvres in children.

with respiratory compromise of sudden onset associated with coughing, gagging and stridor.

Infants

Back blows and chest thrusts are recommended for the relief of foreign body obstruction; abdominal thrusts are not used because of the risk of causing intra-abdominal injury.

• *Back blows.* The infant is placed along one of the rescuer's arms in a head-down position. The rescuer then rests their arm along their thigh, and delivers five back blows with the heel of their free hand (Fig. 11.11).

• *Chest thrusts.* The infant is placed supine along the rescuer's thigh in a head-down position. One hand is used to support the head and five chest thrusts are given using the other hand. The same landmarks as for cardiac compression in this age group are used but at a slower rate than if performing cardiac compressions. The mouth is then checked for any foreign objects.

Following these manoeuvres, the airway is reassessed and if spontaneous ventilation is absent an attempt at expired-air ventilation is made.

INFANT BACK BLOWS

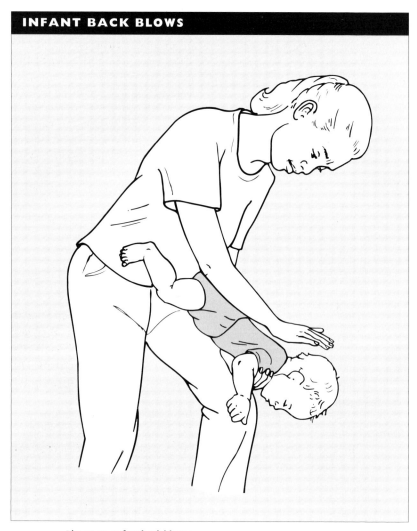

Fig. 11.11 Infant back blows.

Children

Five back blows can be used as for infants. In the older child the Heimlich manoeuvre can be used.

Abdominal thrusts (the Heimlich manoeuvre)

This is performed as in an adult, with the victim standing, sitting or kneeling. It may be necessary for an adult to stand the child on a box or chair, etc. to carry out the standing manoeuvre effectively.

One hand is formed into a fist and placed against the child's abdomen above the umbilicus and below the xiphisternum. The other hand is placed over the fist, and both hands are thrust sharply upwards into the abdomen. This is repeated five times unless the object causing the obstruction is expelled before then.

In a supine child, the rescuer either kneels at their feet, or if the child is large it may be necessary to kneel astride them. The heel of one hand is placed above the umbilicus and below the xiphisternum. The rescuer's other hand is placed over the first, and both hands are thrust sharply upwards into the abdomen, directing the thrust in the midline. This is repeated five times unless the object causing the obstruction is expelled to a point where the patient can cough it out or it can be removed with a finger.

If the child remains apnoeic, ventilation must be attempted before repeating these manoeuvres.

Adult advanced life support

The patient who has collapsed as a result of a cardiorespiratory arrest has the best chance of survival if a spontaneous circulation is rapidly re-established. As the heart most frequently arrests in VF, survival is maximized by early and effective defibrillation which may also be accompanied by intubation and venous cannulation; skills which have already been covered in other chapters.

VENTRICULAR FIBRILLATION

VF is the commonest arrest dysrhythmia and may be preceded by a period of pulseless ventricular tachycardia (VT). The most effective treatment of *both conditions* is identical—electrical defibrillation (a DC shock). The time to delivery of the first shock is critical in determining the outcome, and therefore defibrillation is the first manoeuvre to be carried out in ALS. The only exception to this is when it is preceded by a precordial thump. This manoeuvre should only be used if the cardiac arrest was witnessed and/or monitored. A sharp blow is delivered to the patient's sternum with a closed fist, which effectively delivers a small amount of mechanical energy to the myocardium and if early enough after the onset of VF, may cause the rhythm to revert to one capable of restoring the circulation.

DEFIBRILLATION

Electrical defibrillation or cardioversion depolarizes a critical mass of the myocardium allowing the natural pacemaker of the heart to take over and restore a normal co-ordinated contraction. Defibrillators consist of a power source, either mains or battery, which charges a capacitor to a predetermined level. This energy is discharged through specially designed electrodes or 'paddles' placed on the patient's chest wall. In adults, the paddles are usually 13–14 cm in diameter. To reduce the resistance between paddles and the chest wall, defibrillator pads are used and the paddles applied with firm pressure. The paddles are placed anterolateral: one to the right of the sternum, just below the clavicle; and the other over the apex, below and to the left of the nipple. Although the paddles are marked positive and negative, each can be placed in either position (Fig. 11.12). An alternative is to place them anteroposterior to the heart.

Safety

The discharge of a defibrillator delivers enough current to cause as well as to treat VF. Therefore the user must ensure that neither they nor other rescuers are in contact with the patient or trolley, directly or indirectly (via spilt electrolyte solution), when the defibrillator is discharged. This is usually achieved by clearly shouting 'stand back' and then checking the area visually. Once the defibrillator is charged, the paddles must either be in place on the patient's chest or resting in the defibrillator. Finally, care must be taken to ensure that the paddles are not touching when on the chest, or connected by over-liberal application of electrode gel as this will cause arcing on discharge, insufficient current being delivered and the patient being burned. In addition to the electrical hazards, remove any nitrate patches or ointment (Percutol) to prevent explosions!

> The safety of the resuscitation team is the responsibility of the person carrying out defibrillation.

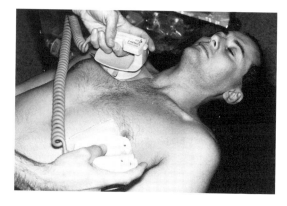

Fig. 11.12 Paddle position for external cardiac defibrillation. Courtesy of Greaves I, Hodgetts T, Porter K. *Emergency Care—A Textbook for Paramedics.* London: Harcourt Brace, 1997.

Technique of defibrillation

1   Turn on the power switch.
2   Ensure the synchronization switch is set to 'OFF'.
3   Select the appropriate energy.
4   Press the charge button.
5   Apply either electrode gel or pads to the chest wall.
6   When machine indicates fully charged, remove the paddles and place in position with firm pressure.
7   Shout 'stand back' and visually check the area and the monitor.
8   Deliver the shock by pressing discharge buttons on both paddles simultaneously.
9   Leave the paddles on the chest if a subsequent shock is to be delivered quickly, or return to the defibrillator if recharging is slow.

> DO NOT HOLD BOTH PADDLES IN ONE HAND WAVING THEM ABOUT!

Synchronized defibrillation

In VF, an unsynchronized shock is delivered, but if an attempt is made to cardiovert ventricular tachycardia, then the shock is best delivered co-ordinated with the 'r' wave, i.e. synchronized. If the shock is delivered on the 't' wave when the heart is refractory, then VF may be precipitated.

Adrenaline

This is a naturally occurring catecholamine, administered during CPR for its profound α-agonist (vasoconstrictor) properties. This leads to an increase in the peripheral vascular resistance which tends to divert blood flow to the vital organs (heart, brain). The adult dose is 1 mg intravenously, i.e. 1 ml of 1:1000 or 10 ml of 1:10 000, administered during ALS every 1–2 minutes. If intravenous (i.v.) access cannot be obtained, larger doses (2–3 mg) can be administered via an endotracheal tube.

OTHER ARREST DYSRHYTHMIAS

Asystole

This represents electrical standstill of the heart with no contractile activity and is seen on the electrocardiogram (ECG) as a gently undulating baseline. Before the diagnosis of asystole is made, it is important to rule out the possibility of VF having been misdiagnosed. This may be due to equipment failure or misinterpretation, for example an ECG lead disconnection, or the gain set too low. If there is any doubt about the diagnosis, treatment should begin as for VF. The risks of not treating VF are greater than that of three unnecessary shocks. A precordial thump can be used under the same criteria as for VF. The outcome is poor unless there are still 'p' waves present.

Electromechanical dissociation

Electromechanical dissociation (EMD) is the term used to describe the situation when there are recognizable regular complexes on the ECG but the patient is pulseless. It is usually a result of conditions which mechanically restrict cardiac filling or outflow, or an acute biochemical disturbance. Common causes are listed in Table 11.3.

> Resuscitation should not, however, be withheld while these conditions are sought, instead they must be eliminated, or if found, treated appropriately whilst resuscitation is in progress.

The patient in EMD should be intubated and i.v. access gained urgently. Adrenaline is administered in the appropriate dose, along with continuous BLS. During treatment of one of the secondary causes, consideration can be given to the use of vasopressors, high-dose adrenaline (5 mg), and calcium chloride. The outcome is poor (< 5%) unless a secondary cause can be found and treated promptly.

Open chest cardiac compression

The output generated by direct compression of the heart is two to three times greater than closed chest compression and coronary and cerebral perfusion pressures are significantly higher. The procedure is performed via a left thoracotomy through the fourth or fifth intercostal space. It is of most use following penetrating trauma, but unlikely to benefit those where cardiac arrest follows blunt trauma. It can also be considered in

CAUSES OF EMD
Hypovolaemia
Tension pneumothorax
Cardiac tamponade
Pulmonary embolus
Drug overdose
Electrolyte imbalance
Hypothermia

Table 11.3 Some common causes of electromechanical dissociation (EMD).

those patients in whom closed chest compression is less effective, namely severe emphysema, a rigid chest wall, severe valvular heart disease or recent sternotomy. There is no evidence to support its use as a routine procedure.

Further reading

European Resuscitation Council. *Guidelines for Resuscitation*. European Resuscitation Council, Antwerp, 1996.

Kouwenhoven WB, Jude JR, Knickerbocker GG. Closed chest cardiac massage. *Journal of the American Medical Association* 1960; **173**: 1064–7.

Safar P, Brown TC, Hotley WH *et al.* Ventilation and circulation with closed chest cardiac massage in man. *Journal of the American Medical Association* 1960; **176**: 574–6.

Index